Healthy Heart

**Strengthen Your
Cardiovascular System**

Healthy Heart

Strengthen Your Cardiovascular System

David Hoffmann
B.Sc., F.N.I.M.H.

STOREY
BOOKS
Schoolhouse Road
Pownal, Vermont 05261

*The mission of Storey Communications is to serve our customers
by publishing practical information that encourages
personal independence in harmony with the environment.*

This publication is intended to provide educational information for the reader on
the covered subject. It is not intended to take the place of personalized medical
counseling, diagnosis, and treatment from a doctor or trained health professional.

Edited by Deborah Balmuth
Cover design by Meredith Maker
Cover art production and text design by Betty Kodela
Text production by Jennifer Jepson Smith and Susan Bernier
Illustration on page 44 by Alison Kolesar; other illustrations by Beverly Duncan,
    Mallory Lake, Sarah Brill, Bobbi Angell, and Brigita Fuhrmann
Indexed by Jon Lewis, Editype

Printed in the United States by Versa Press
10 9 8 7 6 5 4 3 2 1

Library of Congress Cataloging-in-Publication Data

Hoffmann, David, 1951–
        Healthy heart: strengthen your cardiovascular system / David Hoffmann.
        p. cm. — (A Storey medicinal herb guide)
        Includes index.
        ISBN 1-58017-251-2
        1. Herbs — Therapeutic use.   2. Heart — Diseases — Alternative treatment.
        3. Heart — Diseases — Prevention.   I. Title.   II. Medicinal herb guide
        RC684.H47 H64 2000
        616.1'2 — dc21   00-038793

CONTENTS

Introduction: Why Use Herbal Remedies
for Heart Health? 1

1 Minimizing Major Risk Factors 8
General Factors 9
Stress and Personality 13
Cholesterol 14
Dietary and Supplement Guidelines 20

2 Understanding How Herbs Work 23
Herbal Actions for the Heart and More 23
Cardiac Remedies 26
Diuretics 30
A Technical Discussion of Plant Constituents 36

3 Overview of Cardiovascular Diseases 43
Hypertension (High Blood Pressure) 43
Arteriosclerosis 55
Congestive Heart Failure 62
Angina Pectoris 66
Intermittent Claudication 69
Poor Circulation 71
Varicose Veins 73

4 A Guide to the Healing Herbs 78

Arnica • Bugleweed • Cayenne • Cleavers • Coleus • Corn
Couchgrass • Cramp Bark • Dandelion • Feverfew • Figwort
Garlic • Gentian • German Chamomile • Ginger • Ginkgo
Hawthorn • Horsechestnut • Kava Kava • Kola • Lavender
Lily of the Valley • Linden • Lobelia • Ma Huang • Milk Thistle
Motherwort • Night-Blooming Cereus • Oats • Parsley
Passionflower • Prickly Ash • Rosemary • Scots Broom
Siberian Ginseng • Skullcap • St.-John's-Wort • Valerian
Wild Carrot • Witch Hazel • Wood Betony • Yarrow

5 Making Herbal Medicine 109

Teas 110
Tinctures 113
Dry Herb Preparations 114

Index 116

INTRODUCTION
Why Use Herbal Remedies for Heart Health?

When touched by the beauty of a spring meadow in bloom or the profound sense of presence felt in a grove of redwood trees, the heart figuratively takes flight and the spirit is healed. But nature brings physical healing as well, offering nourishment and strength for our troubled hearts.

Half of the annual deaths in the United States result from heart and blood vessel diseases. Herbs offer promise in preventing and easing the symptoms of these diseases. While modern cardiology seems to perform miracles when it comes to treating acute emergencies, such as heart attacks, maintaining good health and preventing the development of disease are critically important. Can we do more for ourselves than simply exercise and minimize risk factors? The answer is an emphatic yes! This is where herbal medicine comes in.

HOW HERBS SUPPORT THE HEART

Herbs have actually held a central position in orthodox medicine for treating various heart problems. Plant constituents called *cardiac glycosides,* which are found in plants such as foxglove and lily of the valley, are used throughout the world for the treatment of heart failure and some arrhythmias. These herbs address these conditions by helping to increase the strength of the heart beat and normalize the rate of the beat. Their real value lies in the increased efficiency they bring to the heart muscle without requiring an increase in the oxygen supply. (In heart problems there is often a deficiency in blood supply — and thus in oxygen supply — because of blockage in the coronary arteries.) Foxglove has this valuable action, although it is also potentially quite toxic. Lily of the valley shares foxglove's therapeutic value but has fewer side effects and lower toxicity. However, there are other herbal remedies that nurture the heart in deeper and more subtle ways. Consider the cordial, a warming drink and a word for heart-felt friendliness. The original cordial was a medieval drink made from borage that warmed the heart and gave a person *heart.*

There are profound concerns about toxicity from the long-term use of prescription medications. Although it is resplendent in "wonder drugs," the modern pharmacopoeia sorely lacks preventive medicines. Tonics are not mentioned in pharmacology texts since the concept of a preventive medicine is illusory. The practice of discarding gentle toning therapies in favor of intensely active ones can be seen as one of the core problems of orthodox health care. This is where herbal medicine can complement and support the orthodox approach — by offering gentle toning therapies. There is a place for this approach alongside the often dramatically successful techniques of cardiology.

Beneficial Actions

A broad range of herbs can be used for the cardiovascular system. As a group, these herbs are known as *cardiac remedies.* Some of these herbs, such as foxglove, are powerful cardioactive agents. Others, such as hawthorn and linden flowers, are gentler and safer cardiotonics.

Cardioactive agents owe their effects to active substances, such as cardiac glycosides. Cardiotonics have a beneficial action on the heart and blood vessels but do not contain cardiac glycosides. The cardiotonics do not have the dramatic, rapid, and often life-saving effects of many cardioactive drugs, but they have an advantage when used to treat or prevent chronic degenerative conditions. Tonics can be used for the blood vessels as well as the heart. These tonics are often rich in constituents called *flavones,* and they include hawthorn, garlic, linden, and ginkgo.

Limitations of Herbal Therapy

Of course, there are some limitations to the use of herbs in treating the heart. The most crucial one today is not an herbal limitation but a human one. The problem, to put it simply, is self-diagnosis: It's a practice that's very hazardous to your health. In the hands of a competent clinical herbalist, medicinal plants offer a great deal for the treatment of cardiovascular conditions. But for the nonprofessional, self-selection of herbs or self-diagnosis can never replace competent diagnosis. Nor can it be a substitute for prescription medicines.

There is a need for safe, effective, readily available and affordable herbs that also have a pleasant taste or aroma or, as the medieval herbalist Gerald would say, are "toothsome." Traditional herbalism offers a cornucopia of remedies that the fit the bill (although, unfortunately, they are not all toothsome!). Such tonic herbs should be part of a holistic program designed to meet the unique needs and circumstances of each individual.

HAWTHORN: A MODEL HERBAL HEART TONIC

Later, I'll discuss the wide variety of herbs used to treat problems of the heart. But it's worth taking a moment to look at one of the most useful herbs for heart health in some detail, as a way of illustrating just how powerful herbal medicine can be.

Hawthorn is the most significant tonic for the heart. The berries and flowers of hawthorn have traditionally been used as cardiac tonics for angina, hypertension, arrhythmias, and congestive heart failure. Stronger herbs are available, but none provides the nourishing regeneration of hawthorn. The late nineteenth-century physician Dr. Ellingwood wrote of hawthorn: "it is superior to any of the well known and tried remedies at present in use for the treatment of heart disease, because it seems to cure while other remedies are only palliative at best."

Hawthorn strengthens the heart in the face of the struggles and strife of life. It is remarkably free of side effects, effective in its actions, and affordable. After a report issued by the German Federal Ministry of Health, hawthorn gained recognition as a heart remedy in Europe (Ammon and Handel. *Planta Medica,* 1981; 43:209). Scientists have found that hawthorn increases the strength of contractions of the heart muscle, normalizes irregular heartbeat, and increases coronary circulation by dilating the coronary arteries. Most significant, no side effects were noted in the studies.

Active Constituents

The primary cardioprotective activity of hawthorn is generally attributed to its flavonoid and oligomeric proanthocyanidin (OPC) content. Although numerous flavonoid molecules have been found to have positive effects on the cardiovascular system, the combination of flavonoid-based constituents in hawthorn seems to provide the beneficial cardiovascular activity.

Many herbal medicines, including ginkgo, bilberry, and milk thistle, owe their physiologic activity to their flavonoid content. Flavonoids have been shown to increase collagen cross-linking in the tissue of vascular walls, strengthen blood vessels, and exert potent antioxidant activity. Recent epidemiologic studies have found an association between dietary flavonoid intake and reduced risk for heart disease, heart attack, and stroke. Flavonoids from hawthorn have been shown to increase coronary blood flow, decrease oxygen consumption by the heart muscle, and reduce coronary spasm. Hawthorn also increases the pumping action of the heart and reduces heart rate.

How Hawthorn Works

How do the berries of this hedgerow bush achieve such results? By dilating the coronary arteries and improving coronary circulation, hawthorn reduces the likelihood of angina attacks and relieves symptoms. It also aids in the availability and utilization of biochemical energy by heart tissue. The result is a gentle but sustained positive effect on degenerative age-related changes. Hawthorn does not produce rapid results, but the results are persistent once they're achieved. To put it simply, hawthorn will help keep the heart healthy by preventing the development of coronary disease. It may be safely used as part of treatment protocols for conditions such as heart failure, angina, and hypertension.

In more technical terms, hawthorn's cardiovascular effects appear to be due primarily to its inotropic and chronotropic effects, enhanced blood vessel integrity, and effects on coronary blood flow and oxygen utilization. It has been suggested that the cardioprotective activity of hawthorn may be due to radical scavenging and inhibition of an enzyme, human neutrophil elastase, by the oligomeric proanthocyanidins of the leaves and flowers. This enzyme is released by white blood cells in greater amounts under conditions characterized by lack of oxygen, and it may be partly responsible, along with free radicals, for damage to the heart. Hawthorn extracts improve the energy dynamics of the heart muscle in such a way that they exert a protective effect on the myocardium.

Clinical Studies

Because of its positive effects on cardiac function, hawthorn extract has been extensively studied for its effect on congestive heart failure. One multicenter, double-blind study used the commonly accepted classification levels for heart failure formulated by the New York Heart Association (see box). One hundred thirty-six patients with cardiac insufficiency categorized as class II were given a hawthorn extract or placebo for 8 weeks. Of these 136 patients, 129 finished the trial. Cardiac function significantly improved in the hawthorn group over the 8-week period. In the placebo group, however, function progressively deteriorated.

HEART FAILURE CLASSIFICATION LEVELS
(developed by the New York Heart Association)

Class I: No limitation in physical activity.

Class II: Slight limitation of physical activity. Comfort at rest, but ordinary physical activity results in fatigue, palpitation, dyspnea, or angina pain.

Class III: Marked limitation of physical activity. Comfort at rest, but less than ordinary physical activity results in fatigue, palpitation, dyspnea, or angina pain.

Class IV: Inability to carry out any physical activity without discomfort.

In his book *Herbal Medicine*, German physician Rudolf Weiss suggests the following indications for hawthorn:

- "Degeneration of the cardiac muscle or coronary artery disease" (anginal symptoms of coronary artery disease can be treated successfully with hawthorn when it's used long-term).
- Hypertension (primarily to improve cardiac function).
- Weakness of the myocardium after infectious disease.
- Muscular insufficiency in patients requiring digitalis.
- Cardiac arrhythmias, mainly extrasystole and tachycardia.

OTHER IMPORTANT HEART HERBS

Ginkgo is another important heart herb that has an abundance of research revealing many important therapeutic effects. In terms of cardiovascular use, the research shows that ginkgo lowers blood pressure, dilates peripheral blood vessels, and increases peripheral blood flow. In patients with peripheral arterial insufficiency there was an improvement in the ability to walk without pain. In addition to having preventive use, ginkgo has been recommended in the treatment of a number of heart and blood vessel problems, especially those due to vascular insufficiency. It is indicated in both peripheral circulatory insufficiency and cerebral vascular insufficiency. An exciting use is in the treatment of circulatory disturbances due to aging, diabetes, and tobacco.

In addition to the heart tonics, other herbal actions can be helpful for people experiencing symptoms related to heart disease. The relaxing herbs are especially important; they include motherwort, linden, skullcap, and valerian. Circulatory stimulants, such as cayenne, ginger, and prickly ash, increase blood flow, supporting oxygenation of tissue and the elimination of waste. This makes them important for circulatory problems as well as for conditions such as rheumatism.

There are other herbs that should be avoided even though they do not contain cardiac glycosides. Examples are Scots broom and ma huang, both of which stimulate heart activity and raise blood pressure. They are contraindicated in many conditions and should not be considered tonics.

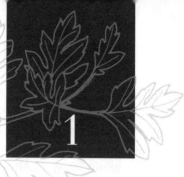

MINIMIZING
MAJOR RISK FACTORS

A well-rounded program to strengthen the heart must involve more than just herbs. There is not enough space here to explore all the other factors in detail, but a major influence on heart disease are risk factors whose effects can be minimized. Whole forests have been turned into paper to print articles about these factors, and anyone trying to read them all and follow the debates that rage is putting him- or herself at risk for a hypertensive crisis!

The origins of heart disease are complex and confusing. Risk factors are habits or traits that make a person more likely to develop a disease. Some risk factors for heart-related problems cannot be changed, but many others can be. The major risk factors that something *can* be done about are cigarette smoking, high blood pressure, high blood cholesterol levels, obesity, and physical inactivity. Other risk factors, such as diabetes, are conditions over which you can exercise some control. Others still, such as age, sex, or heredity, are beyond your control but important for you to understand.

Although widely accepted guidelines for lessening the risk of cardiovascular disease have been developed, simplistic statements linking one specific factor to increased disease incidence can be misleading. For example, one study determined that there was no association between heavy coffee consumption and long-term hypertension. However, the study failed to note that heavy coffee drinkers also tend to be heavy smokers, and heavy smoking may be associated with a lower body weight. Thus, while heavy coffee drinkers may have lower blood pressure, they are also more likely to be at risk of heart attack as a result of the association between coffee and smoking!

GENERAL FACTORS

Having just one of the following risk factors will increase your chances of having heart-related problems. The more risk factors a person has, the more likely he or she is to develop cardiovascular diseases.

Age and Sex Factors

The older a person is, the more likely she or he is to develop cardiovascular disease. The risk of heart attack is four times greater for a 50-year-old man than for a 30-year-old man. Such problems are unusual in premenopausal women, although the incidence in postmenopausal women is the same as that in men.

Oral contraceptives. Birth control pills with high doses of estrogen increase the risk of vascular and heart disease, especially in women who smoke. However, the currently prescribed contraceptives are "low-dose" pills that have 35 micrograms of estrogen or less. Premenopausal women using these contraceptives have little additional risk for heart disease. However, oral contraceptives do pose risks. If you are taking any kind of birth control pill or are considering using one, keep these guidelines in mind:

- Stop smoking or use a different form of birth control. Smoking boosts the risks of serious cardiovascular problems resulting from oral contraceptive use, especially the risk of blood clots. The risk is greatest in women over 35.

- Birth control pills may increase blood pressure.
- If you take birth control pills and are diabetic or prediabetic, you should have your blood sugar tested regularly.
- If you have had problems with blood clots, a heart attack, or a stroke or if you have any other kind of cardiovascular disease, oral contraceptives may not be a safe choice.

Heredity

The tendency to develop a range of cardiovascular diseases seems to be partly inherited. People with a family history of heart disease should do everything possible to offset this risk, including changing their diet, reducing emotional stress, and using herbal tonics.

Diet

The wealth of research done has shown that heart disease has definite links with dietary fat, raised blood cholesterol, raised blood pressure, obesity, short stature, and lack of physical activity. The precise role of these factors is unclear, but enough is known to formulate general dietary guidelines for prevention. These are discussed in more detail on pages 20–22.

Tobacco

The death rate from heart disease in North America is 300 percent higher in smokers than in nonsmokers. In women in the United States, smoking causes 1.5 times as many deaths from heart disease as from lung cancer. A smoker is two to six times more likely to suffer a heart attack than a nonsmoker is, and the risk increases with the number of cigarettes smoked each day. Smoking also heightens the risk of stroke.

Of course, cardiovascular diseases are not the only health risks connected to smoking. Cigarette smoking is also linked with cancers of the mouth, larynx, esophagus, urinary tract, kidney, pancreas, and cervix. Smokers are more likely to develop lung problems other than cancer, including bronchitis and emphysema. Smoking during pregnancy is linked to several problems, including bleeding, miscarriage, premature delivery, lower birthweight, stillbirth, and sudden infant death syndrome (SIDS, or "crib death"). In addition, young children who breathe secondhand smoke have more lung and ear infections. What more needs to be said?

Alcohol

A small amount of alcohol may actually benefit the circulatory system because of its vasodilating effects. Several recent studies have reported that moderate drinkers — those who have one or two drinks per day — are less likely to develop heart disease than people who don't drink any alcohol. However, this is *not* a recommendation to start using alcohol!

Moderation is the key. More than three alcoholic drinks per day can raise blood pressure, and binge drinking can lead to stroke. People who regularly drink heavily have higher rates of heart disease than moderate drinkers or nondrinkers. According to the U.S. government's "Dietary Guidelines for Americans," an individual should consume no more than one drink per day for overall health. One drink equals 12 ounces of beer, 5 ounces of wine, or 1½ ounces of 80-proof liquor.

High Blood Pressure

High blood pressure is a major risk factor for coronary heart disease and is the most important risk factor for stroke and heart failure. It causes three of every five cases of heart failure in women, and it boosts the chances of developing kidney disease and blindness.

Controlling high blood pressure is especially important for people with heart disease. When blood pressure is lowered, the heart doesn't have to work as hard. For example, a person who has had a heart attack is less likely to have another if he or she controls high blood pressure. Blood pressure is considered high when it stays above 140/90 over a period of time (see pages 43–48).

Obesity

Compared with people of normal weight, obese people are more likely to develop heart-related problems, even if they have no other risk factors. Excess body weight is linked to coronary heart disease, stroke, congestive heart failure, and death from heart-related causes. Obesity contributes not only to cardiovascular diseases but also to such risk factors as high blood pressure, high blood cholesterol levels, and diabetes.

Sedentary Lifestyle

Physical inactivity increases the risk of heart disease. It contributes directly to heart-related problems and increases the chances of developing other risk factors, such as high blood pressure and diabetes. The U.S. Surgeon General's report and other current research conclude that as little as 30 minutes of moderate activity on most, preferably all, days of the week is enough to help protect heart health. Examples of moderate activity include brisk walking or bicycling, raking leaves, or gardening. Find a form of exercise that is both aerobic and enjoyable for you.

Diabetes

Diabetes is a serious disorder that increases the risk of coronary heart disease. The risk of death from heart disease is about three times higher in people with diabetes. Although there is no cure for diabetes, you can take steps to control it. In certain people, being overweight and growing older are linked to the development of the most common type of diabetes. Maintaining ideal body weight and boosting physical activity may help postpone or prevent the onset of diabetes.

STRESS AND PERSONALITY

Researchers have shown that the risk of heart disease differs between people with two extreme types of behavior. Those at the highest risk are those with "type A" behavior, which is characterized by a chronic sense of urgency, aggressiveness (which may be repressed), and striving for achievement. People with this personality type drive themselves to meet deadlines, many of which are self-imposed; they have feelings of being under pressure; and they often do two or three things at once. They are likely to react with hostility to anything that seems to get in their way, and they are temperamentally incapable of letting up.

"Type B" behavior is characterized by the opposite traits: being less preoccupied with achievement, feeling less rushed, and generally being more easy-going. People with this type of personality are less prone to anger and do not feel constantly impatient, rushed, or pressured. They are also better at separating work from play, and they know how to relax.

The value of such personality typing is controversial, and the details of this are beyond the scope of this book. The important thing to recognize is the association between certain types of behavior and the development of disease. We also need to remember that there really aren't two distinct types of people: Every person is an individual. While it may sometimes be useful to sort people into artificial categories, these categories do not truly identify the individual.

Socioeconomic Factors

Social and economic factors are associated with an increased risk of heart disease. However, the findings tend to vary according to the society being studied. Some studies have found higher risks in people with higher socioeconomic status, whereas others have found higher risks in people with lower socioeconomic status. Some evidence suggests that class difference is minimized when the degree of physical activity is taken into account. High-risk factors include:

- Social mobility involving a change of environment, such as moving to a new house in a different type of neighborhood or changing jobs and entering a company with a different social atmosphere or structure.
- The relatively low occurrence of heart disease in (premenopausal) women compared with men seems to have some psychosocial causes as well as biological factors. Men are more likely to have an exaggerated striving for dominance and to use work as a major outlet for aggression. As a result, they tend to be more exposed to particular stresses and conflicts that are risk factors for heart disease.

Stressful Life Events

Particularly stressful times in a person's life are potential triggers for angina and heart disease. When these stressful situations are identified and addressed, their effects on health and well-being can be managed and lessened.

CHOLESTEROL

Cholesterol plays a natural part in the body's metabolism. It is the major sterol in the human body and is, in fact, found throughout the animal kingdom. It's in all cells of the human body, primarily as a structural component of cell membranes. It has other vital functions as well. Stored in the adrenal glands, testes, and ovaries, it is converted to hormones such as the sex hormones (androgens and estrogens) and the adrenal corticoids (including cortisol, corticosterone, and aldosterone). In the liver, it is the precursor of the bile acids that are secreted into the intestine to aid in the digestion of food, especially fats.

Cholesterol has been implicated as a major factor in the development of many cardiovascular diseases, especially arteriosclerosis. Arteriosclerosis occurs when fatty deposits accumulate on the linings of large and medium-size arteries. The presence of the fatty deposits, called *plaques*, leads to a loss of elasticity in and a narrowing of vessels. This constriction ultimately deprives organs of their blood supply. Clots may lodge in arteries supplying the heart and cause a heart attack. Or clots may form in the brain, causing a stroke.

Measuring Blood Cholesterol Levels

Blood cholesterol levels generally start rising at about age 20. They increase most sharply beginning at about age 40 and continue to increase until about age 60. The higher an individual's blood cholesterol level, the higher that person's risk of having a heart disease.

In the bloodstream, cholesterol binds with protein molecules to form various types of lipoproteins. High-density lipoprotein (HDL) is a dense, compact microparticle that transports excess cholesterol to the liver, where it is altered and expelled in bile. Low-density lipoprotein (LDL) is a larger, less dense particle that tends to remain in the body. Very-low-density lipoprotein (VLDL) transports triglycerides — chemical compounds that store fatty acids, which are an essential source of energy for the body.

Cholesterol packaged as LDL is often called "bad" cholesterol because too much LDL in the blood can lead to cholesterol buildup and blockages in the arteries. Cholesterol packaged as HDL is known as "good" cholesterol because it helps remove cholesterol from the blood and thus prevents it from piling up in the arteries.

What Do Cholesterol Levels Mean?

A desirable total cholesterol level for adults without heart disease is less than 200 mg/dL (200 milligrams per deciliter of blood). A level of 240 mg/dL or higher is considered to be high. But even levels in the borderline-high category (200–239 mg/dL) increase the risk of heart disease.

HDL levels are interpreted differently. The lower the HDL level, the higher the risk of heart disease.

	Desirable	Borderline-High	High
Total cholesterol	Less than 200	200–239	240 and above
LDL cholesterol	Less than 130	130–159	160 and above

An HDL cholesterol level less than 35 mg/dL is a major risk factor for heart disease. An HDL level of 60 mg/dL or higher is protective.

(Source: Second Report of the Expert Panel on Detection, Evaluation, and Treatment of High Blood Cholesterol in Adults, National Institutes of Health, NHLBI, 1993.)

Lowering Cholesterol Naturally

Diets rich in saturated fats, cholesterol, and calories seem to be chiefly responsible for high blood cholesterol levels and therefore are believed to promote atherosclerosis. However, the plaque-forming tendency of cholesterol is influenced by the type of lipoproteins that transport it in the blood. The LDLs are clearly troublesome, but the HDLs seem to prevent accumulation of cholesterol in the tissues. Blood levels of these lipoproteins are partially governed by dietary factors, especially the type of vegetable lipids (phytosterols) that people eat.

Phytosterols are plant compounds that are structurally similar to cholesterol. They effectively block uptake of cholesterol in the liver. The processes involved are complex and not completely understood. Many common dietary components are revealing themselves to be active in lowering cholesterol levels in the blood. However, how they achieve this is not always known.

Following are some of the natural remedies that seem to show the most promise.

Gugulipid. An herbal remedy from southern India, gugulipid (*Commiphora mukul)* is gaining a reputation for reducing high blood cholesterol levels. It is an extract from a close relative of the myrrh tree, and its ability to control cholesterol and triglyceride levels has been compared to that of some synthetic drugs. It seems to lower LDL and raise HDL levels without causing side effects.

Cayenne pepper. Along with other plants that contain the compound capsaicin, cayenne has a well-demonstrated effect in lowering blood cholesterol levels.

Fenugreek and caraway. These widely used spices have demonstrable cholesterol-lowering properties.

***Emblica officinalis* and *Ligustrum lucidum*.** These are just two of a whole range of Asian herbal remedies that are new to western medicine and are proving to be valuable in this field.

Garlic and onion. Both garlic and onion have international reputations for lowering blood pressure and generally improving the health of the cardiovascular system. One recent study of the effects of consuming garlic was conducted on two groups: The first consisted of 20 healthy volunteers, and the second comprised 62 patients with coronary heart disease and high cholesterol levels. Tracked over a period of ten months, both groups showed improvements in cholesterol levels, which reached a peak at the end of eight months. The improved cholesterol levels persisted throughout two months of clinical follow-up. The clinicians concluded that the essential oil of garlic possesses a distinct hypolipidemic, or fat-reducing, action that benefits both healthy people and those with coronary heart disease.

Researchers in India conducted a clinical study on the influence of garlic on people who eat a diet rich in fats. A group of volunteers were fed a fat-rich diet for 7 days; on the eighth day their fasting blood was analyzed for cholesterol and other fats. They were then fed a fat-rich diet with the addition of garlic for the following 7 days, and on the fifteenth day of the study their fasting blood was analyzed again. The results showed a significant elevation in the cholesterol levels tested on the eighth day but a significant reduction in serum cholesterol levels in the blood tested on the fifteenth day, after garlic had been added to the diet.

Garlic has been shown to reduce the formation of unwanted blood clots within blood vessels. It seems to work on the "stickiness" of blood platelets and inhibit the release of clotting factors in the blood. This is thought to be a property of allicin, a unique thiosulfinate in garlic that is known for its strong antibiotic and antifungal properties. An exciting new finding is that garlic can work selectively. In other words, it inhibits the synthesis of enzymes involved in plaque formation while sparing the vascular synthesis of important prostaglandins. This makes it a safe and effective antithrombotic (or anticlotting) agent.

Because of studies on the effects of raw garlic, many scientists now recommend its daily use for lowering blood cholesterol. Interestingly, garlic's effectiveness in normalizing and lowering cholesterol is not lost as a result of cooking, while its antimicrobial effects do appear to be lost when it is cooked. The traditional use of onions for treating hypertension are also now being supported by research. It was recently found that onion oil contains a blood pressure–lowering agent, prostaglandin.

A Cholesterol–Lowering Plan

A high cholesterol level is a serious risk factor for heart disease. Bringing it down to a healthful point requires a multistep process.

To lower total cholesterol levels along with LDL levels:
- Decrease total fats in your diet.
- Decrease saturated fats in your diet.
- Decrease cholesterol in your diet.
- Increase essential fatty acids (polyunsaturates) in your diet.
- Use more monounsaturated oils, such as olive or canola oil.

- Increase fiber intake.
- Use psyllium husks.
- Add oat bran to your diet.
- Increase your intake of complex carbohydrates.
- Decrease caffeine and nicotine use.
- Take supplements of vitamins B_6, B_3, and C; chromium; eicosapentaenoic acid; and garlic.

To increase HDL cholesterol levels:
- Get regular aerobic exercise.
- Do not smoke.
- Lose weight.
- Take supplements of essential fatty acids, niacin, eicosapentaenoic acid, fiber, garlic, and L-carnitine.

To reduce cholesterol in your diet, try to avoid:
- Egg yolks
- Liver and other organ meats
- Full-fat dairy foods
- Fatty meats
- Palm oil

To reduce saturated fats in your diet, try to avoid:
- Butter
- Full-fat dairy products, including cheese and milk
- Red meats
- Poultry
- Coconut oil
- Avocados
- Margarine

To get more monounsaturated fats in your diet, try to consume more:
- Olives and olive oil
- Almonds, pecans, peanuts, cashews, and walnuts
- Fish

To substitute polyunsaturated fats for saturated fats, use:
- Vegetable oils: sesame, safflower, sunflower, corn, and soybean

DIETARY AND SUPPLEMENT GUIDELINES

A wealth of research in recent years has shown that a healthful diet goes a long way toward reducing the risk of heart disease. The basic dietary rules for lowering cholesterol levels are simple: Avoid saturated fats and dietary cholesterol. Experts recommend a diet in which no more than 30 percent of daily calories comes from fat — no more than 20 percent might be even better. Saturated fats derived from animal products and tropical oils should be kept to a minimum, so avoid eating deep-fried foods. Pay attention to the nutrition labels on packaged foods. Eat more vegetables, fruits, and grains, which are cholesterol-free, almost fat-free, and rich in fiber.

- Eat food that you like that is also low in cholesterol and the saturated fats. A diet free of animal products is one of the best ways to lower cholesterol levels and blood pressure.
- Get plenty of dietary fiber. Two of the best sources of fiber are oat bran and psyllium seeds.
- Minimize salt, avoid stimulants, and drink little or no alcohol.
- Eat more fruits and vegetables.
- Eat more whole grains.
- Reduce fat intake to 25 to 30 percent of total calories.
- Reduce cholesterol intake to less than 300 mg per day.
- Reduce consumption of egg yolks to three to five per week.
- Minimize use of whole milk and other full-fat dairy foods.
- Avoid red meats, including cured meats and lunchmeats.
- Eat more cold-water fish, such as sardines and salmon.
- Use fresh, cold-pressed oils, such as olive or flaxseed oils, which provide essential fatty acids.

Coenzyme Q_{10}

Coenzymes are molecular cofactors upon which enzymes depend for their function. Coenzyme Q_{10}, also called *ubiquinone*, is found in small amounts in a wide variety of foods and is synthesized in all tissues of the body.

Coenzyme Q_{10} is required for many mitochondrial enzymes, as well as enzymes in other parts of the cell. Mitochondria are small, subcellular particles responsible for energy production. They contain electron transport chains, which are the fundamental units for energy production in the cells. Mitochondrial enzymes are essential for the production of adenosine triphosphate, upon which all cellular functions depend. More than 95 percent of the oxygen we breathe is used solely for making energy through this process.

Other substances involved in this electron transport chain include vitamin C, riboflavin (vitamin B_2), niacinamide (vitamin B_3), vitamin E, and others. Coenzyme Q_{10} plays a unique role: It is a mobile messenger link between the various enzymes of the chain. Each pair of electrons processed by the chain must first interact with coenzyme Q_{10}. No other substance can be substituted for it.

A wide variety of foods contain coenzyme Q_{10}, but the following are particularly high in this substance: organ meats, such as heart, liver, and kidney; beef; soy oil; sardines; mackerel; and peanuts. To put dietary coenzyme Q_{10} into perspective, you'd have to eat 1 pound of sardines, 2 pounds of beef, or 2½ pounds of peanuts to get 30 mg of coenzyme Q_{10}.

Even though coenzyme Q_{10} is present in food, it is not considered a vitamin because the body can make it from raw materials contained in food. Nevertheless, the body often cannot make enough for optimal functioning. Therefore, coenzyme Q_{10} supplements may be very helpful.

Coenzyme Q_{10} is highly concentrated in heart muscle cells because of their high energy requirements. Congestive heart failure has been correlated with low blood and tissue levels of coenzyme Q_{10}. The severity of heart failure correlates with the severity of coenzyme Q_{10} deficiency, and this deficiency may well be a primary factor in some types of heart muscle dysfunction and a secondary phenomenon in other types.

Whether primary, secondary, or both, this deficiency of coenzyme Q_{10} seems to be a major treatable factor in the otherwise inexorable progression of heart failure. Clinical studies of treatment of heart disease with coenzyme Q_{10} have concluded that it significantly improves heart muscle function while producing no adverse effects or drug interactions. Coenzyme Q_{10} has been used successfully to treat high blood pressure, congestive heart failure, angina pectoris, and cardiomyopathy. It has also been shown to protect the heart from the damaging effects of the chemotherapeutic drug adriamycin.

Homocysteine

Homocysteine is an amino acid normally found in the body. High blood levels of homocysteine may increase the chances of developing heart disease, stroke, and circulation problems. It is thought that elevated homocysteine levels damage the arteries, predispose the blood to easy clotting, and reduce the flexibility of blood vessels.

Blood homocysteine levels are inversely related to three vitamins in the diet: folic acid, vitamin B_6, and vitamin B_{12}. Ingesting less than the recommended daily amounts of these vitamins may lead to higher homocysteine levels. The daily amounts of these nutrients recommended by the U.S. Food and Drug Administration are 400 micrograms folic acid; 2 mg vitamin B_6; and 6 micrograms vitamin B_{12}. Good sources of folic acid include citrus fruits, tomatoes, vegetables, whole grains, beans, and lentils. Foods high in vitamin B_6 include meat, poultry, fish, fruits, vegetables, and grains. Major sources of vitamin B_{12} are meat, poultry, fish, milk, and other dairy products.

2

UNDERSTANDING
HOW HERBS WORK

Extensive pharmaceutical research has analyzed the active constituents of herbs to find out how and why they work. However, a much older and far more relevant approach is to categorize herbs not by their active constituents but by the kinds of problems they have successfully been used to treat. In some cases, the action is due to a specific chemical present in the herb. In other cases, it may be due to a complex synergistic interaction among various constituents of the plant rather than one particular constituent.

HERBAL ACTIONS
FOR THE HEART AND MORE

To be a well-educated consumer of herbal medicine, you need to understand the vocabulary herbalists use to describe the primary actions that herbs exhibit. While some of these words are probably familiar to you, others may not be. This vocabulary list is worth learning because you'll see these terms used repeatedly throughout this book and in other health-related literature.

Even though specialists in herbal medicine have an enormous variety of healing herbs to choose from, most herbs for protecting the cardiovascular system are *cardiac remedies*, *diuretics*, or *hypotensives*. These terms, along with many others, are defined in the following list. Why include those that do not seem to apply to cardiovascular health? Because herbs are complex and often have more than one action. Thus, an herb that is a cardiac remedy may also be an astringent. It's important to understand all of the properties of a given herb before you use it.

Adaptogen. Increases resistance and resilience to stress, enabling the body to adjust to the problem. Adaptogens seem to work by supporting the adrenal glands.

Alterative. Gradually restores proper functioning of the body, increasing health and vitality. Some alteratives support natural waste elimination through the kidneys, liver, lungs, or skin. Others stimulate digestive function or are antimicrobial, and others just work!

Anticatarrhal. Helps the body remove excess mucus in the sinuses or other parts of the body. Mucus itself is not a problem, but too much mucus may be produced in response to an infection or as a way for the body to get rid of excess carbohydrates.

Anti-inflammatory. Soothes or reduces inflammation. These herbs work in many different ways, but they rarely inhibit the natural inflammatory reaction directly. Rather, they support the body as it is working.

Antimicrobial. Helps the body destroy or resist pathogenic microorganisms. Some herbs have antiseptic properties, but antimicrobials generally work by strengthening the body's natural immunity.

Antispasmodic. Eases muscle cramps and helps relieve muscular tension. Many antispasmodics are also nervines, and these also relieve psychological tension.

Astringent. These have a bracing action on mucous membranes, skin, and other tissue. Because of chemicals called *tannins,* astringents bind with protein molecules, reducing irritation and inflammation and creating barriers against infections. These herbs are helpful for healing wounds and burns.

Bitter. Bitter-tasting herbs have a special role in preventive medicine. The taste triggers a sensory response in the central nervous system, and this causes the intestine to release digestive hormones. Bitters are used to stimulate the appetite and the flow of digestive juices. They also aid the liver in detoxification, increase bile flow, and stimulate self-repair mechanisms in the gut.

Cardiac remedy. This is a general term for herbal remedies that have a beneficial action on the heart. Some cardiac remedies are powerful cardioactive agents, such as foxglove; others are gentler, safer herbs, such as hawthorn and motherwort.

Carminative. Stimulates the digestive system, soothes the gut wall, reduces inflammation, eases griping pains, and helps remove gas from the digestive tract.

Demulcent. Soothes and protects irritated or inflamed tissue. These herbs reduce irritation down the whole length of the bowel, reduce sensitivity to potentially corrosive gastric acids, and help prevent diarrhea. They also reduce the muscle spasms that cause colic along with the bronchial tension that causes coughing.

Diaphoretic. Promotes perspiration and thus helps the skin eliminate waste from the body. Some diaphoretics produce observable sweat, while others aid normal perspiration. They often promote dilatation of surface capillaries, which improves circulation. They support the work of the kidneys by increasing cleansing through the skin.

Diuretic. Increases the production and elimination of urine. In herbal medicine, with its ancient traditions, the term is often applied to herbs that have a beneficial action on the urinary system as a whole. Diuretics help the body eliminate waste and support the process of inner cleansing.

Emmenagogue. Stimulates menstrual flow and activity. The term is also applied to remedies that normalize and tone the female reproductive system.

Expectorant. Stimulates removal of mucus from the lungs and acts as a tonic for the respiratory system. Stimulating expectorants "irritate" the bronchioles, causing expulsion of material. Relaxing expectorants soothe bronchial spasms and loosen mucus secretions, thereby relieving dry, irritating coughs.

Hepatic. Aids the liver by toning; strengthening; and, in some cases, increasing the flow of bile. These herbs are important because of the liver's fundamental role in the body.

Hypotensive. Lowers abnormally elevated blood pressure.

Laxative. Stimulates bowel movements. Laxatives should not be used long term; diet, general health, and stress levels should all be closely considered when constipation persists.

Nervine. All three types of nervines help the nervous system. Nervine tonics strengthen and restore the nervous system, nervine relaxants ease anxiety and tension by soothing both body and mind, and nervine stimulants directly stimulate nerve activity.

Rubefacient. Generates a localized increase in blood flow when applied to the skin, thereby encouraging healing, cleansing, and nourishment. These herbs are often used to ease the pain and swelling of arthritic joints.

Tonic. Nurtures and invigorates. Tonics truly are gifts from nature to a suffering humanity. To ask how they work is to ask how life works!

Vulnerary. Promotes wound healing. Used mainly to describe herbs that heal skin lesions. Vulneraries also work for internal wounds, such as stomach ulcers.

CARDIAC REMEDIES

Cardiac remedy is a general term for herbal remedies that benefit the heart. Some of these remedies are powerful cardioactive agents, such as foxglove, while others are gentler and safer cardiotonics, such as hawthorn and linden.

In a strictly technical sense, the pharmacological term *cardiotonic* refers to an herb that increases the strength of the heart muscle's contractions, the frequency of beats, the volume of beats, or cardiac performance in general.

In the herbal literature, the definitions of these terms are different. The two groupings of herbs that prove most useful in clinical practice are as follows:

- **Cardioactive**. These are plants that contain cardiac glycosides or other very active substances and thus have both the strengths and drawbacks of these constituents.
- **Cardiotonic.** These plants have an observable, beneficial action on the heart and blood vessels but do not contain cardiac glycosides. The way in which cardiotonic herbs work is obscure and a matter of pharmacologic debate. The following research review offers some insights.

How Cardioactive Remedies Work

Cardioactive remedies owe their power to the presence of the cardiac glycoside group of plant constituents, which increase the efficiency of the muscles of the heart without increasing their need for oxygen. This enables the heart to pump enough blood around the body without causing a buildup of fluid in the lungs or extremities. This sounds wonderful, and it is, but there is always the possibility of accruing too much of the glycosides in the body, as the

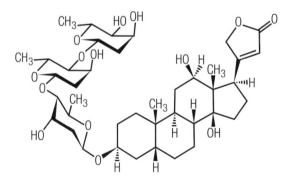

Digoxin, a cardiac glycoside in foxglove, helps increase the efficiency of the muscles of the heart without increasing their need for oxygen. However, too much digoxin is potentially poisonous.

removal rate tends to be low. This effect is the main drawback of foxglove and is why it is potentially poisonous if it isn't used with skill and knowledge. Clinically trained medical herbalists often use lily of the valley rather than foxglove because lily of the valley is associated with a smaller risk for such problems.

Benefits of Cardiotonics

Cardiotonics have been shown to have beneficial actions on the heart and blood vessels, but exactly how they work is a subject of scientific debate. Flavones seem to be major contributors to the beneficial role of these tonic remedies, which include hawthorn, linden, garlic, and motherwort.

Pharmacologists around the world are searching for plants with cardiovascular activity. They are seeking not simply herbs and new constituent compounds with the potency of the cardiac glycosides, but also substances that may be useful for adjuvant heart therapy, geriatric heart conditions, or milder cardiac insufficiency. This research involves a variety of approaches for selecting herbs for testing and a recognition of the value of herbal traditions. It has identified various cardiotonic substances, including the phenylalkylamines found in the night-blooming cereus; alkaloids, such as those in prickly ash and Scots broom; and the flavonoids in hawthorn and bilberry.

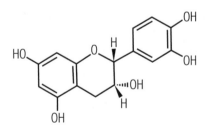

Epicatechin, a flavonoid found in hawthorn.

Cardiotonics for Various Parts of the Body

When an herb has such a specific action, it is not usually relevant to all body systems. However, many cardiotonics do affect parts of the body other than the heart and blood vessels. Following are some examples:

- **The circulatory system.** Remedies that primarily have cardioactive effects on circulation include lily of the valley, foxglove, Scots broom, squill, figwort, and bugleweed. The tonic remedies include hawthorn, linden, garlic, and motherwort. Remedies that specifically benefit the blood vessels are hawthorn, linden, horsechestnut, garlic, ginkgo, and yarrow.
- **The respiratory system.** Any condition affecting the heart may also cause lung congestion because of the backlog of blood waiting to be pumped. The cardiac tonics may indirectly benefit the lungs by helping the heart. Garlic is renowned for its antimicrobial effects as well as its beneficial actions on the lungs. Angelica is another gentle cardiac tonic that will help with lung problems.
- **The digestive system.** Several herbs for the heart, including rosemary, linden, motherwort, yarrow, angelica, garlic, and balm, also support the digestive system.
- **The urinary system**. Most of the herbs that directly aid the heart's action will increase the amount of blood passing through the kidneys. As a result, they act as diuretics. Yarrow is an herb used in urinary problems, as is Scots broom.
- **The reproductive system.** The cardiotonics do not directly involve the functioning of the reproductive system. Yarrow may play a dual role, but it affects the reproductive system only very slightly.
- **The muscular and skeletal systems.** Herbs that act as circulatory stimulants affect the entire body and often play an important role in the musculoskeletal system by increasing peripheral blood flow. They are sometimes used to reduce swelling and ease stiffness. Such herbs include cayenne, ginger, prickly ash, mustard, and horseradish.

- **The nervous system.** Motherwort, linden, balm, and rosemary all have a relaxing effect on the nervous system. As we shall see, many nervines help the circulatory system by relaxing the mind and body as a whole.
- **The skin.** The only directly relevant remedy here is figwort. However, for skin problems due to varicosity in the veins, cardiotonics such as hawthorn, horsechestnut, linden, and yarrow are very important.

DIURETICS

Diuretics are therapeutic agents that help the body rid itself of excess water by increasing the rate of urine production by the kidneys. The accumulation of excess fluids in tissues, known as *edema*, is a symptom of a wide range of heart, kidney, liver, and other disorders.

Diuretics may be used with other herbs. Many diuretics alter the excretion of electrolytes by the kidneys. The electrolytes, such as sodium and potassium salts, are involved in many body processes, including the regulation of blood pressure, nerve impulse transmission, and muscle contraction.

In herbal medicine, the term *diuretic* has come to imply herbs that have some sort of beneficial action on the urinary system, not merely herbs that remove excess fluids from the body. Thus, the term has come to be applied to urinary demulcents and anti-inflammatory remedies. This expanded definition can, regrettably, lead to confusion when remedies are being selected for a particular person. The following discussion should clarify this situation to some degree.

How Diuretics Work

If we limit ourselves to the strict sense of the term *diuretic*, there seem to be two broad groups: Diuretics that increase blood flow in the kidneys, and diuretics that reduce water reabsorption in the nephrons of the kidneys.

The first group includes not only diuretics such as Scots broom but also all herbs that are cardioactive, such as foxglove, and circulatory stimulants. Because they cause more blood to pass through the kidneys, more urine is produced. Caffeine-containing herbs, such as kola, guarana, tea, and coffee, also have this effect.

The second group works in many different ways. These herbs cause diuresis because some of their constituents are secreted by the kidneys. This may change the osmotic balance, causing the body to lose more water. Dandelion leaf, couchgrass, and cornsilk are three herbs that seem to work in this way. Others in this group work by irritating the reabsorption mechanism in the kidneys through volatile oils, saponins, or alkaloids such as uva-ursi.

IMPORTANT DIURETIC HERBS

Agrimony (Agrimonia eupatoria)

Bearberry (Arctostaphylos uva-ursi)

Boneset (Eupatorium perfoliatum)

Buchu (Barosma betulina)

Bugleweed (Lycopus europaeus)

Celery seed (Apium graveolens)

Cleavers (Galium aparine)

Corn silk (Zea mays)

Couchgrass (Elytrigia repens ssp. repens)

Dandelion leaf (Taraxacum officinale)

Elderleaf (Sambucus nigra)

Gravel root (Eupatorium purpureum)

Hawthorn (Crataegus species)

Kola (Cola acuminata)

Lily of the valley (Convallaria majalis)

Linden (Tilia species)

Parsley (Petroselinum crispum)

Scots broom (Cytisus scoparius)

Sea holly (Eryngium maritimum)

Stone root (Collinsonia canadensis)

Wild carrot (Daucus carrota)

Yarrow (Achillea millefolium)

Other Herbs with Diuretic–Like Properties

Some herbs have a markedly diuretic impact, and others primarily affect the kidneys. For example, it's possible to reduce inflammation by using demulcents and anti-inflammatories. Infections can be treated directly with "diuretics" that are mainly antimicrobial. Similarly, when problems are associated with kidney stone formation, the herbalist may choose plants known as *antilithics*, which help the body rid itself of kidney stones or gravel.

Groups of herbs with diuretic-like properties include the following:

- **Anti-inflammatory.** Celery seed, cleavers, corn silk, couchgrass, gravel root.
- **Antilithic.** Gravel root, hydrangea, stone root.
- **Antimicrobial.** Bearberry, buchu, couchgrass, juniper, yarrow.
- **Astringent.** Agrimony, bearberry, broom, horsetail, kola, yarrow.
- **Demulcent.** Bearberry, corn silk, couchgrass, stone root.

Secondary Actions of Diuretics

Each herb has a range of actions apart from its primary effects on a specific body system or organ. The urinary system and diuretics are fundamental to many bodily functions. The secondary actions and system affinity of the diuretic herbs are important to understand. For example, diuretic herbs may affect body systems other than the urinary system in the following ways:

- **The circulatory system.** As we've seen, the cardioactive remedies have a diuretic effect because they increase blood flow through the kidneys. These herbs include lily of the valley, Scots broom, dandelion, and yarrow. Care should be taken to ensure that the right herbs are used for the specific condition being treated. For example, Scots broom should not be used to lower high blood pressure as it constricts the small blood vessels in the body, leading to a rise in blood pressure.

- **The respiratory system.** If pulmonary congestion is resulting from heart problems, most of the diuretics will be of value. Remedies that have an affinity for the respiratory system include boneset, cleavers, elder, eucalyptus, and yarrow.
- **The digestive system.** Some of the laxative herbs also act as diuretics; these include agrimony, blue flag, boldo, borage, celery seed, dandelion, parsley, and pumpkin seed.
- **The reproductive system.** The antiseptic diuretics are often helpful for the reproductive system. Bearberry has special relevance as it is an effective antimicrobial diuretic. Saw palmetto is a mild diuretic.
- **The muscular and skeletal systems.** Because of their cleansing action, many diuretics help alleviate problems of muscles and bones. These herbs include boneset, celery seed, gravel root, and yarrow.
- **The nervous system.** Borage and bugleweed are the only real diuretics that directly affect the nervous system. However, if there is much tension, use of a nervine may allow more urine to be passed.
- **The skin.** All the diuretics potentially help the skin by an inner cleansing process. Especially notable are cleavers, couchgrass, and dandelion. An important point is that some diuretics act as diaphoretics when they are drunk hot.

The following list notes the secondary actions of some specific diuretic herbs.

- **Anticatarrhal.** Boneset, elder.
- **Anti-inflammatory.** Borage, celery seed, cleavers, gravel root.
- **Antimicrobial.** Bearberry, buchu, couchgrass, juniper, saw palmetto, yarrow.
- **Astringent.** Agrimony, bearberry, broom, bugleweed, cleavers, horsetail, kola, yarrow.

- **Bitter.** Agrimony, burdock.
- **Cardioactive.** Broom, bugleweed, lily of the valley.
- **Demulcent.** Bearberry, corn silk, couchgrass, parsley piert, pellitory of the wall, stone root.
- **Diaphoretic.** Boneset, borage, elder, linden, yarrow.
- **Emmenagogue.** Parsley, yarrow.
- **Expectorant.** Borage, elder, parsley.
- **Galactogogue.** Borage.
- **Hepatic.** Boldo.
- **Hypotensive.** Hawthorn, linden, yarrow.
- **Laxative.** Boneset.
- **Nervine.** Bugleweed, celery seed, kola, linden.
- **Tonic.** Agrimony, boneset, buchu, cleavers, dandelion, saw palmetto.

HYPOTENSIVE HERBS

Hypotensive herbs are useful for reducing elevated blood pressure, tending to normalize both systolic and diastolic pressures. These include the following herbs:

Black cohosh *(Cimicifuga racemosa)*

Black haw *(Viburnum prunifolium)*

Buckwheat *(Fagopytum esculentum)*

Cramp bark *(Viburnum opulus)*

Fenugreek *(Trigonella fenugraecum)*

Garlic *(Allium sativum)*

Hawthorn berries *(Crataegus laevigata)*

Linden *(Tilia* species)

Mistletoe (European) *(Viscum album)*

Motherwort *(Leonurus cardiaca)*

Nettles *(Urtica dioica)*

Onion *(Allium cepa)*

Parsley *(Petroselinum crispum)*

Passionflower *(Passiflora incarnata)*

Siberian ginseng *(Eleutherococcus senticosus)*

Skullcap *(Scutellaria laterifolia)*

Valerian *(Valeriana officinalis)*

Vervain *(Verbena officinalis)*

Yarrow *(Achillea millefolium)*

SECONDARY ACTIONS OF HYPOTENSIVES

Following are the secondary actions of specific hypotensive herbs.

Adaptogen: Siberian ginseng.

Alterative: Black cohosh, garlic.

Anticatarrhal: Fenugreek, garlic, onion.

Anti-inflammatory: Black cohosh, buckwheat, valerian.

Antimicrobial: Garlic, onion, yarrow.

Antispasmodic: Black cohosh, black haw, cramp bark, garlic, linden, motherwort, passionflower, skullcap, valerian, vervain.

Astringent: Black haw, cramp bark, linden, nettles, yarrow.

Bitter: Yarrow.

Cardiotonic: Buckwheat, hawthorn berries, motherwort.

Carminative: Parsley, valerian.

Cholagogue: Garlic, vervain.

Demulcent: Fenugreek.

Diaphoretic: Garlic, linden, onion, vervain, yarrow.

Diuretic: Linden, nettles, parsley, yarrow.

Emmenagogue: Black cohosh, motherwort, parsley.

Expectorant: Fenugreek, garlic, onion, parsley.

Galactagogue: Fenugreek.

Hepatic: Onion, vervain.

Laxative: Vervain.

Nervine: Black cohosh, black haw, cramp bark, linden, mistletoe (European), motherwort, passionflower, skullcap, valerian, vervain.

Tonic: Black cohosh, buckwheat, fenugreek, garlic, hawthorn berries, nettles, onion, skullcap.

Vulnerary: Buckwheat, fenugreek, onion.

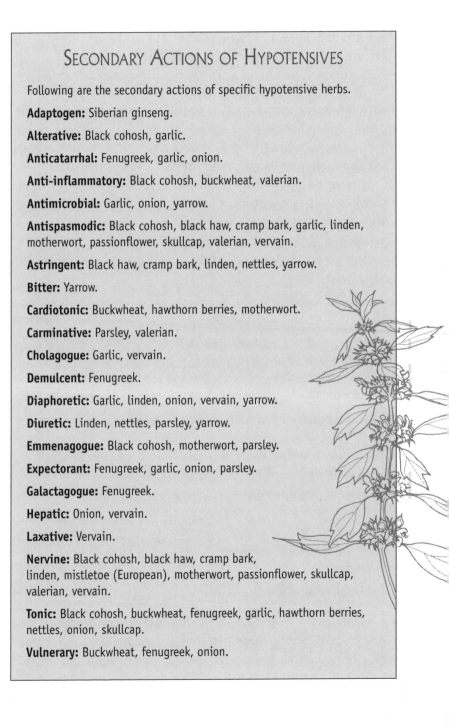

A TECHNICAL DISCUSSION OF PLANT CONSTITUENTS

This more technical section is offered to indicate the depth of scientific attention that herbal remedies are now receiving from medical researchers, and to provide some of the research results for interested readers. We shall briefly discuss effects on the heart itself and then broader effects on the cardiovascular system.

There are a range of ways in which a substance may affect the activity of the heart. Below is a list of these actions and the characteristic actions of compounds of plant origin. Some classes of substances, like the cardiac glycosides and the sympathomimetics, appear several times as they exert several different types of activity on the heart.

ACTIVITY	DEFINITION	CONSTITUENT
Positive inotropic	Increase of contractility	Cardiac glycosides
Negative inotropic	Decrease of contractility	ß-blockers
Positive chronotropic	Increase of cardiac frequency	Sympathomimetics
Negative chronotropic	Decrease of cardiac frequency	Cardiac glycosides
Positive dromotropic	Increase of flow rate	Sympathomimetics
Negative dromotropic	Decrease of flow rate	Cardiac glycosides
Antiarrhythmic	Removal of cardiac arrhythmia	Quinidine
Coronary dilating	Dilation of coronary arteries	Flavonoids, theophylline

Cardioactive and Cardiotonic

As discussed in the earlier section on cardiac remedies (see pages 26–30), the pharmacological term *cardiotonic* is synonymous with *positive inotropic*. However, *cardiotonic* is also used to indicate an increase in frequency, an increase in beat volume, or a general increase in cardiac performance, in addition to increased contraction. In the herbal literature slightly different terms are used. The two groupings that prove most useful in clinical practice are:

- **Cardioactive plants** owe their effects on the heart to cardiac glycosides or other very active substances and thus have both the strengths and drawbacks of these constituents.
- **Cardiotonic plants** have an observably beneficial action on the heart and blood vessels but do not contain cardiac glycosides. The way they work is either completely obscure or is an area of pharmacological debate. The research reviewed below offers some insights.

Cardiac Glycosides

Cardioactive remedies, as we discussed earlier, owe their properties to cardiac glycosides, which have the unique effect of increasing the heart's efficiency without increasing its need for oxygen. This lets the heart pump enough blood around the body while ensuring that there is no buildup of fluid in the lungs or extremities. However, there is always the possibility of accruing too much of the glycosides in the body, as their solubility and removal rates tend to be low. This is the main drawback of foxglove and is the reason why it can be poisonous if not used with skill and knowledge.

Cardiac glycosides occur in plants in two structural forms, the cardenolides and bufanolides. Cardenolides are the most common and are particularly abundant in the Dogbane and Milkweed families. However, they are also found in some lilies, such as lily of the valley, and in the Buttercup, Fig, Mustard, Cacao, Spurge, Bittersweet, Pea, and Figwort families. The bufanolides occur in some members of the Lily family, such as squill, and in some Buttercup relatives.

The overall action of the *digitalis* glycosides is complicated by the number of different effects produced, and their exact mode of action on myocardial muscle is still an area of investigation. *Digitalis* probably acts in competition with potassium ions for specific receptor enzyme (ATPase) sites in the cell membranes of cardiac muscle and is particularly successful during the depolarization phase of the muscle when there is an influx of sodium ions. The clinical effect in cases of congestive heart failure is to increase the force of contraction. The diuretic action of *digitalis* arises from the improved circulatory effect.

Nonsteroid, Cardioactive Plant Constituents

The observation that consumption of fruits and vegetables shows an inverse relationship with heart disease in epidemiological studies cannot be explained by vitamins, minerals, and macronutrients alone. A recent review of the literature highlights evidence that phytosterols, flavonoids, and plant sulfur compounds lower the risk of cardiovascular disease (Howard and Kritchevsky. *Circulation*, 1997;95:2591–2593).

In the search for potential cardioactive compounds, a number of approaches are used to select herbs for pharmacological testing.

- Reinvestigation of old literature reports of cardiac activity.
- Investigation of plants used in "folk medicine."
- Selection of plants from families that have other cardioactivities.
- Search for chemical types already known to possess potential cardiac activity.

This has led to the identification of eight main classes of nonsteroidal cardiotonic substances: phenylalkylamines, indole derivatives, tetrahydroisoquinolines, imidazoles and purines, diterpenes, sesquiterpenes, flavonoids, and other phenolic compounds. Here we shall briefly focus on those found in the primary cardiovascular herbal remedies.

Although orthodox medicine makes much use of cardioactive agents of plant origin, the search for new active substances with a better therapeutic picture and with different or new types of activity continues. This active field of research is bringing a number of plants to the attention of practitioners. In addition to noting plants such as hawthorn and garlic, research highlights other remedies new to the west. For example *Polygonatum sibiricum* is an active cyclic adenosine monophosphate (AMP) phosphodiesterase inhibitor, the effect correlating with strength of heart muscle contraction. The isolation of forskolin from the roots of *Coleus forskohlii* shows that plants offer western medicine new and potent cardiac agents. The diterpene forskolin is an unexpected cardioactive compound, displaying a specific activation of adenylate cyclase.

Although considered to be the "active ingredient," many other diterpenoids have been reported (DeSouza and Shah. In *Economic and Medicinal Plant Research.* London: Academic Press; 1988). Forskolin lowers blood pressure and in small doses it has a positive ionotropic effect. Topical ocular application of forskolin lowers intra-ocular pressure. Forskolin reduces preload and afterload of the heart through its vasodilating action, and it augments myocardial contractility because of its positive inotropic action without affecting myocardial oxygen consumption.

Phenalkylamines

This class of plant constituents was the model for the development of sympathomimetic drugs. The main representative is L-ephedrine, first found in ma huang (*Ephedra sinica*). Since ephedrine has other more prominent activities, its action on the heart is considered a side effect. Ephedrine and its relatives have been found in many plants in a wide range of families. The plants include numerous food plants, such as citrus fruits, bananas, and purslane. Synephrine occurs in the fruit of the mandarin orange.

Cathinone, from Khat, shows strong positive inotropic activity, contributing to the well-known cardiac stimulation activity of Khat leaves.

Phenylethylamines are widely distributed, occurring in the Cactaceae, Rosaceae, Rutaceae, and Leguminosae. Strong positive inotropic activity is displayed by N-methyltyramine, hordenine, and p-methoxy-phenethylamine, all of which have been found in hawthorn flowers. Phenylethylamines are also found in night-blooming cereus, a remedy for cardiac insufficiency and angina pectoris.

Other Nitrogen–Containing Compounds

Cardiotonic activity is found in certain alkaloids. Alkaloids from the bark of Amazonian bush *Cymbopetalum brasiliense* act synergistically and are at least partly responsible for the herb's positive inotropic activity. Methylcanadine from prickly ash and sanguinarine from blood root also possess positive inotropic activity. The lupine alkaloid sparteine possesses specific antiarrhythmic activity. Cyclic AMP also possesses inotropic properties and is widely distributed in plants.

Phytosterols

Phytosterols have been shown to lower blood cholesterol levels by 10 percent, possibly by inhibiting cholesterol absorption. Plasma cholesterol decreases were possibly due to increased low-density lipoprotein (LDL) receptor activity.

Plant Sulfur Compounds

The *Allium* genus contains sulfur compounds that may influence plasma cholesterol. A meta-analysis of garlic suggests that the consumption of half a garlic clove per day lowers serum cholesterol by 9 percent. Garlic is thought to inhibit cholesterol synthesis.

Flavonoids

Several large population studies show an inverse relationship between the consumption of flavonoids and coronary heart disease. The Zutphen Elderly Study found a coronary heart disease mortality rate of 18.5 per 1000 person-years for people who consumed 0 to 19.0 mg per day of flavonoids. People who consumed more than 29.9 mg per day of flavonoids had a mortality rate of 7.8 per 1000 person-years. Five to six cups of tea would contain approximately 29.9 mg of flavonoids. Some flavonoids possess antioxidant qualities that inhibit LDL oxidation. Flavonoids have been shown to inhibit platelet aggregation and adhesion, a process by which arteries become blocked. Comprehensive investigations and reviews have been published on the cardioactivity of *Crataegus*, as discussed below. The main active principles are thought to be flavonoids and procyanidin oligomers. The evidence suggests that the flavonoids exert their cardiotonic action by inhibition of cellular phosphodiesterase and elevation of the cellular cyclic AMP concentration, as well as by affecting the permeability of cell organelles to calcium ions. This inhibitory activity towards phosphodiesterase is not limited to flavonoid structures. A series of lignans were also potential phosphodiesterase inhibitors.

Hypotensives

In orthodox medicine today, synthetic ß-blockers, ACE-inhibitors, and calcium-channel blockers play an essential role in the treatment of hypertension. Intensive research over many years has revealed plants that possess some of the activity of these drugs. Here we shall consider the calcium-channel blockers. Calcium-antagonistic drugs are widely used in the treatment of cardiovascular disorders such as angina pectoris, myocardial infarction, atherosclerosis, and hypertension. Even though the currently used calcium-channel blockers have different chemical structures and sites of action, it is established that they inhibit the influx of calcium ions across the membrane through "voltage-dependent calcium channels." This reduces smooth-muscle contractility and vascular resistance, resulting in a lowering of the blood pressure.

The main therapeutic influence is on the function of heart and circulation of the blood. Hypotensives are coronary dilators; they reduce peripheral vascular resistance and hence reduce the cardiac workload. Furthermore, they are energy-sparing drugs that slow the rate of ATP exhaustion. The three main groups of prescription calcium-channel blockers are dihydropyridines, benzodiazepines, and phenylalkylamines. They include common compounds used in therapy, such as nifedipine, diltiazem, and verapamil.

Calcium–Channel Blockers Detected in Plants

The impetus to search for calcium-channel blockers in plants is motivated by the following considerations. Traditional medicine in various countries possesses numerous plants with antihypertensive, vasodilatory, spasmolytic, or diuretic activity, but for most of them the mode of action is unknown. Yet in recent years, various plant constituents have shown apparent calcium-channel blocking activity in some in vitro screening models. A recent review of calcium antagonists isolated from plants suggests that many have activity comparable to that of compounds currently used in therapy and are considered worth examining further.

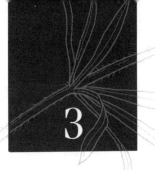

OVERVIEW OF CARDIOVASCULAR DISEASES

Cardiovascular diseases are disorders of the heart and blood vessels. Coronary heart disease, for example, is a disease of the blood vessels of the heart, which are known as *coronary arteries*. Coronary heart disease causes chest pain (angina) and heart attacks.

Blood brings oxygen and nutrients to the heart. When too little blood flows to the heart, angina results. When blood flow is critically reduced, a heart attack occurs. A similar event may occur in the brain. A lack of blood flow to the brain or, in some cases, bleeding in the brain, causes a stroke. Another cardiovascular disease is high blood pressure (hypertension), which is discussed in the following section.

HYPERTENSION (HIGH BLOOD PRESSURE)

Blood travels through the body by flowing through blood vessels called *arteries,* carrying oxygen from the heart to other tissues and organs. Once the oxygen is delivered to the tissues and organs, oxygen-poor blood travels back to the heart through veins. The heart then pumps this blood into the lungs, where it is replenished with oxygen. After returning to the heart, the blood is pumped out into the arteries again.

Blood pressure is the force exerted by blood against artery walls as it circulates through the body. The body monitors and adjusts blood pressure through a complex interaction among the heart, blood vessels (both arteries and veins), nervous system, kidneys, and several hormones, in response to various stimuli.

More than 35 million people in the United States have hypertension, and twice as many cases occur among African Americans as among Caucasians. The reasons for this difference are not known. A common problem in western societies, hypertension is rare in cultures that are relatively untouched by the western lifestyle. Dietary, psychological, social, and other lifestyle factors must be addressed for any real change in the incidence of hypertension in western culture.

Measuring Blood Pressure

The Circulatory System

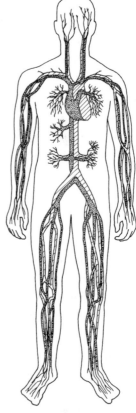

This diagram shows the network of veins (dark areas) and arteries (striped areas) that make up the human circulatory system.

Each time the heart beats, about 60 to 70 times a minute in normal circumstances, it pumps blood into the arteries. Blood pressure is at its greatest when the heart contracts to pump the blood. This stronger pressure is called *systolic pressure*. When the heart is at rest in between beats, the blood pressure falls. This lower pressure is called *diastolic pressure*.

Blood pressure is measured in fractions of millimeters of mercury (mm Hg) by means of a special instrument called a sphygmomanometer. It has an inflatable rubber cuff attached to a pressure-monitoring device. The two numbers that indicate your blood pressure are expressed as a fraction, for example 120/80 mm Hg. The first number is the systolic pressure (when the heart contracts to pump blood through the arteries); the second number is the diastolic pressure (when the heart relaxes and fills with blood for the next contraction).

When blood pressure is measured in a doctor's office, the cuff is placed around the arm and pumped up with air to momentarily stop the circulation of blood. As the pressure inside the cuff is reduced, blood begins to flow again. The person measuring the blood pressure uses a stethoscope to the sounds the blood makes as it flows through the arteries. By listening closely to these sounds and noting on the sphygmomanometer the exact numbers at which they start and stop, one can measure the systolic and diastolic pressures.

A blood pressure reading of less than 140/90 mm Hg is considered normal; a blood pressure below 120/80 mm Hg is even better. (See the chart on page 46 for a complete detailing of classification ranges for blood pressure levels in adults.) It used to be thought that low blood pressure (e.g., 105/65 mm Hg in an adult) was unhealthy. Except in rare cases, this is not true.

Disorders Affecting the Heart

Generalized Cardiovascular Disorders
- Hypertension
- Hypotension
- Arteriosclerosis
- Atherosclerosis

Diseases of the Heart
- Congestive heart failure
- Myocardial ischemic disorders
- Angina pectoris
- Myocardial infarction
- Cardiomyopathies
- Valvular heart disease

Peripheral Vascular Disorders
- Intermittent claudication
- Raynaud's phenomenon
- Thrombosis
- Varicose veins

CLASSIFICATION OF BLOOD PRESSURE LEVELS IN ADULTS*		
CATEGORY	SYSTOLIC	DIASTOLIC
Normal	120	80
High Normal	130–139	85–89
High/Stage 1	140–159	90–99
High/Stage 2	160–179	100–109
High/Stage 3	≥180	≥110

*For people who are not taking medicine for high blood pressure and do not have a short-term serious illness.

Causes

As discussed in chapter 1, there are several risk factors that may contribute to whether or not an individual develops hypertension. Some of these, such as weight, diet, and lifestyle, are risk factors you can control. Consumption of alcoholic beverages and smoking, which cause blood pressure to rise, are examples of risk factors you have the power to eliminate. Other risk factors, such as age, heredity, race, and gender, cannot be changed.

Some fluctuations in blood pressure are normal and result from various activities. When people are physically active, for example, blood pressure naturally rises. During sleep, blood pressure goes down. Such changes are normal and healthy. However, some people have blood pressure that stays high most of the time. This consistent elevation can lead to serious medical problems if it isn't treated.

Symptoms

Hypertension typically has no symptoms until complications arise. The symptoms associated with the condition include dizziness, flushing, headache, fatigue, epistaxis (nose bleeding), and nervousness. A doctor can also detect high blood pressure by looking at changes in the blood vessels in the retinas.

Serious Complications

If high blood pressure is not treated and lowered, it can lead to any of the following complications:

- **Arteriosclerosis.** High blood pressure changes the artery walls, making them thick and stiff. This speeds the buildup of cholesterol and fats in the blood vessels, inhibiting blood flow through the body and increasing the risk of heart attack or stroke.
- **Heart attack.** Blood carries oxygen to the body. When the arteries that bring blood to the heart muscle become blocked, the heart cannot get enough oxygen. Reduced blood flow can cause chest pain (angina). Eventually, the flow may be stopped completely, causing a heart attack (also called a *myocardial infarction*).
- **Enlarged heart.** High blood pressure makes the heart work harder. Over time, the heart thickens and stretches. Eventually, the heart fails to function normally, and this causes fluids to back up into the lungs. Controlling high blood pressure can prevent this.
- **Kidney damage.** The kidneys act as filters to rid the body of wastes. Over many years, high blood pressure can narrow and thicken the blood vessels of the kidneys. The kidneys then filter less fluid, and wastes build up in the blood. As a result, the kidneys may fail altogether.
- **Stroke.** High blood pressure can cause arteries to narrow, decreasing blood flow to the brain. If a blood clot blocks one of the narrowed arteries, a stroke may occur. A stroke can also occur when very high pressure causes a rupture in a weakened blood vessel in the brain.

It's important to differentiate between elevated blood pressure with no obvious medical cause (primary or essential hypertension) and elevated blood pressure that is due to an underlying abnormality, such as kidney, endocrinological, or cerebral disease (secondary hypertension). The discussion in this chapter is concerned with essential hypertension. A temporary increase in blood pressure is a common and normal response to the ups and downs of life. Sustained hypertension is caused by increased peripheral vascular resistance. This is initiated by increased arteriolar tone and then followed by structural changes of arteriosclerosis.

Herbs for Hypertension

Any specific herbal treatment plan or list of herbal remedies for a condition reflects wisdom and experience gained through study and long-term observation of the effects of various herbs. These remedies should not be considered a substitute for a balanced prescription that takes individual needs into account.

That said, the herbal treatments that may be considered for hypertension include the following:

- **Hypotensives.** These are used to lower high blood pressure. They seem to work in a variety of ways, including through most of the actions described for the other entries in this list. Examples of hypotensive herbs include garlic, hawthorn, and cramp bark.
- **Cardiac tonics.** These play a fundamental role in strengthening and toning the whole cardiovascular system. Used correctly, they facilitate beneficial changes in both the pattern and the volume of cardiac output. The most relevant example of a cardiac tonic is hawthorn.

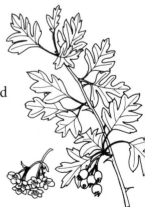

- **Vasodilators.** These lessen high resistance within the peripheral blood vessels, increasing the total volume of the system and lowering the pressure within it. Hawthorn, cramp bark, and ginkgo should be considered.
- **Diuretics.** These help remove excessive buildup of water in the body and overcome any decrease in renal blood flow that may accompany hypertension. Mild diuretics usually suffice. Diuretics that also have appropriate tonic properties are yarrow, hawthorn, and linden.
- **Vascular tonics.** These nourish the tissues of the arteries and veins. Again, yarrow, hawthorn, and linden come to mind.
- **Relaxing nervines.** These address the tension and anxiety associated with any stress caused by hypertension. They also reduce the muscle tension caused by the hypertension itself. Examples include motherwort and skullcap.
- **Antispasmodics.** These alleviate peripheral resistance to blood flow by gently relaxing both the muscles that the vessels pass through and the muscular linings of the vessels themselves. Cramp bark and valerian are two examples.
- **Circulatory stimulants.** These may help increase peripheral circulation.

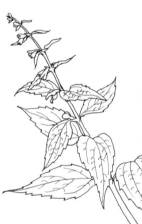

A number of herbs have a reputation for being specific for hypertension, usually working by having an impact on one or more of the processes that contribute to the development of the condition. The hypotensive herbs fit this description. The most important herbal remedy for hypertension in the western tradition is hawthorn, followed by linden. European mistletoe and olive leaves are other specific remedies often used. However, because there are so many factors that contribute to the development of hypertension, it is not particularly valuable to seek one specific treatment.

Hypertension Formula

This combination of herbs includes hypotensives (hawthorn, linden blossom, yarrow, cramp bark, valerian), cardiac tonics (hawthorn, linden blossom), diuretics (yarrow, hawthorn, linden blossom), antispasmodics (linden blossom, cramp bark, valerian), vascular tonics (hawthorn, linden blossom, yarrow), and nervine relaxants (linden blossom, cramp bark, valerian).

2 parts hawthorn 1 part yarrow
1 part linden blossom 1 part cramp bark

To make: Combine herbs and make a tincture as directed on pages 113–114.
To use: Take ½ teaspoon (2.5 mL) three times per day. In addition, take 2 capsules of garlic oil daily with food.

Stress-Related Hypertension Formula

If stress is a contributing factor to hypertension, use the following formula, which has increased nervine content.

2 parts hawthorn 1 part skullcap
1 part linden blossom 1 part cramp bark
1 part yarrow 1 part valerian
1 part Siberian ginseng

To make: Combine herbs and make a tincture as described on pages 113–114.
To use: Take ½ teaspoon (2.5 mL) of the tincture three times per day. In addition, take 2 capsules of garlic oil daily with food.

Hypertension with Headache Formula

If headaches are part of the experience of hypertension, including wood betony can be beneficial.

> 2 parts hawthorn
> 1 part linden blossom
> 1 part yarrow
> 1 part cramp bark
> 2 parts wood betony

To make: Combine herbs and make a tincture as described on pages 113–114.

To use: Take ½ teaspoon (2.5 mL) of the tincture three times per day. In addition, take 2 capsules of garlic oil daily with food.

Formula for Hypertension-Related Palpitations

For cases of hypertension accompanied by heart palpitations, motherwort can be a beneficial addition.

> 2 parts hawthorn
> 1 part linden blossom
> 1 part yarrow
> 1 part motherwort
> 1 part cramp bark
> 1 part valerian

To make: Combine herbs and make a tincture as described on pages 113–114.

To use: Take ½ teaspoon (2.5 mL) of the tincture three times per day. In addition, take 2 capsules of garlic oil daily with food.

A Broader Perspective on Hypertension

A plethora of factors has been identified as important in understanding the cause and treatment of essential hypertension. However, it must be remembered that causation always involves a range of factors and that citing a single factor, such as alcohol or calcium, is often too simplistic and ignores related factors. For example, as discussed earlier, one study found no association between heavy coffee consumption and long-term hypertension. Heavy coffee drinkers, however, tend to be heavy smokers as well, and this in turn may be associated with a lower body weight and thus a lower blood pressure. But coffee and smoking combined present an increased risk of heart attack!

Dietary factors may have a strong correlation with hypertension. The primary factors to consider include:

- **Dietary sodium.** Average salt intake in the western world is about 15 times greater than what the body needs. A low-salt diet is strongly indicated. Usually, blood pressure decreases if people with high blood pressure cut back on sodium intake. Some people are more affected by sodium than others. Because there is no practical way to predict who will be affected, it makes sense to limit sodium intake to help prevent high blood pressure.

  People with high blood pressure should eat no more than about 6 g of salt per day (about 2400 mg of sodium, or 1 teaspoon of table salt). Remember to keep track of all salt consumed, including the salt in processed foods and the salt added during cooking or at the table.
- **Potassium.** The relative balance between sodium and potassium is crucial for many people. In addition to restricting salt intake, it's helpful to increase dietary potassium levels by eating potassium-rich foods, such as bananas, and by using cooking methods that do not wash this essential mineral away.

- **Calcium and magnesium.** Supplementation with these minerals can have a significant pressure-lowering effect. Supplement the diet with magnesium (800 to 1200 mg per day), vitamin C (500 to 1000 mg three times per day), vitamin E (400 to 800 IU per day), coenzyme Q10 (50 mg two to three times per day), and garlic (the equivalent of 4000 mg per day, fresh).
- **Obesity.** The link between obesity and hypertension is well known; obesity also contributes to heart attack, diabetes, gallstones, osteoarthritis, and kidney disease. Weight reduction is essential for obese people, and it often lowers blood pressure more effectively than drug treatment.
- **Sugar.** In some people, heavy sugar intake may raise blood pressure, possibly by causing sodium retention or by affecting the body's stress-response hormone system.
- **Alcohol.** There appears to be a link between alcohol and hypertension, but it's not a simple one. Statistics show that people who drink a little alcohol tend to have lower blood pressure than teetotalers or those who drink a lot. However, alcohol withdrawal temporarily increases blood pressure. It's probably safe to say that people at risk for hypertension should avoid alcohol.
- **Caffeine.** Tea, coffee, and cola drinks aggravate hypertension because of the stimulating effects of the caffeine and other alkaloids that they contain.
- **Tobacco.** Experts disagree about the connection between tobacco and hypertension. However, there is no disagreement about the effect of smoking on overall heart health. People who smoke should make every effort to quit.
- **Saturated fats.** There seems to be an association between high levels of saturated fat intake and hypertension, and this association is quite separate from the effects of saturated fats on cholesterol levels. As with all cardiovascular conditions, increasing the ratio of polyunsaturated fats to saturated fats will help the healing process.

- **Vegetarian diet.** A diet free of animal products definitely lowers blood pressure and is strongly advised for hypertensive patients. At the very least, avoid red meat.
- **Drugs.** Many medications raise blood pressure as an unwanted side effect. Check all prescription drugs and note that even over-the-counter medications, such as ibuprofen, may cause mild water retention that can elevate blood pressure.
- **Oral contraceptives.** Controversy still rages over the side effects of the Pill. One area of debate is the Pill's hypertensive effects. If you're taking oral contraceptives or plan to do so, discuss the possibility of side effects with your doctor.

KEY DIETARY AND LIFESTYLE THERAPIES FOR HYPERTENSION

- Maintain an appropriate body weight, reducing excessive weight if necessary.
- Eliminate salt from the diet.
- Make healthy lifestyle choices. Avoid alcohol, caffeine, and tobacco.
- Reduce the impact of stress. Exercise regularly but in a way that is enjoyable to you.
- Eat a diet rich in fiber, complex carbohydrates, and potassium.
- Eat garlic and onions.
- Reduce or eliminate animal fats and increase intake of vegetable oils.
- Supplement the diet with:
  Magnesium: 800–1200 mg daily
  Vitamin C: 500–1000 mg three times a day
  Vitamin E: 400–800 IU daily
  Coenzyme Q$_{10}$: 50 mg 2–3 times a day
  Garlic: the equivalent of 4000 mg per day of fresh garlic

Other Lifestyle Factors

Lifestyle can often be the key to reversing high blood pressure. The nature of the individual's work, relationships, world view, and self image may all contribute to hypertension, making it challenging to identify the varied factors and select the most appropriate herbs to address these concerns. Techniques that may help control hypertension include:

- Exercise
- Massage
- Other bodywork therapies
- Aromatherapy — hypotensive essential oils to consider include lavender, marjoram, and ylang-ylang. For relaxation, oils such as chamomile and rose may be used.

CALL YOUR DOCTOR IF:

- You experience side effects such as drowsiness, constipation, dizziness, or loss of sexual function when taking antihypertensive medications.

- You are pregnant and develop hypertension.

- You have severe headaches, nausea, blurred vision, or confusion.

- Your diastolic pressure (the second figure in your blood pressure reading) rapidly rises to more than 130.

ARTERIOSCLEROSIS

The term *arteriosclerosis* refers to several diseases that involve arteries of different sizes, as well as different layers of the walls of the arteries. The term comes from Greek words that mean "hardening of the arteries." Hardening of the arteries is not, however, an important characteristic of the most familiar form of arteriosclerosis, called *atherosclerosis*.

Although some herbs may have anti-arteriosclerotic properties, herbalism primarily aims to prevent the disease by addressing its underlying causes, among them hypertension, diabetes, smoking, and obesity.

Understanding Atherosclerosis

Atherosclerosis is a disease of the arteries that is characterized by the formation of fatty deposits on the inner lining of the arteries. The presence of fatty deposits, called *plaques*, leads to an important loss of arterial elasticity. It also narrows the inside of the artery. This narrowing is what ultimately deprives vital organs of their blood supply. Clots may lodge in plaque-filled arteries supplying the heart, causing a heart attack. Or, the clots may form in arteries in the brain, causing stroke.

Atherosclerosis is so prevalent in developed countries that many Americans assume it is a natural consequence of aging. However, overwhelming evidence links atherosclerosis closely to diet and lifestyle, and this suggests that atherosclerosis can be prevented or slowed — even, in some cases, reversed.

Depending on the location and the degree of arterial damage, atherosclerosis can cause kidney problems, high blood pressure, stroke, and other life-threatening conditions. Atherosclerosis tends to target the aorta — the body's largest artery — as well as arteries leading to the brain, lower limbs, and kidneys.

Damage to arteries carrying blood to the legs and feet makes walking painful; in severe cases, restricted circulation to the limbs can cause skin ulcers and even gangrene (tissue death). Blockage in the coronary arteries, which feed oxygen-rich blood directly to the heart muscle, is known as *coronary artery disease*. This disorder and its complications — angina, arrhythmias (irregular heartbeat), and heart attack — are leading causes of death in the United States and most of Europe.

Disease Progression

The deposits begin as thin, fatty streaks on an arterial wall. Such streaks may come and go in a person with a healthy lifestyle. If the arteries are damaged — typically as a result of high blood pressure, stress, or smoking — the inner surfaces of the walls can start to deteriorate. To compensate, the artery grows new tissue. This creates tiny bumps or scars. Cholesterol, white blood cells, and other deposits can start to accumulate within these bumps, forming plaques that clog the arteries. Eventually, calcium deposits and scar tissue surround the soft plaque, making the arteries hard and inelastic.

Atherosclerosis progresses over many years, and this contributes to the fact that it is perceived as an affliction of aging. However, arterial deposits can begin in childhood, and significant plaque formation can have occurred by the time a person is 30.

Risk Factors

People with high levels of blood cholesterol, especially low-density lipoprotein (LDL) cholesterol, are at risk for atherosclerosis. LDL cholesterol reacts with unstable molecules called *free radicals*. This process degrades the transport mechanisms for moving cholesterol through the bloodstream and the tissues lining arterial walls. Nonetheless, most people with high cholesterol levels do not develop atherosclerosis, and many people with atherosclerosis have normal cholesterol levels.

Half the annual mortality rate in western society results from heart and blood vessel diseases, of which atherosclerosis, the most lethal common disease, is the chief cause because of its impact upon the brain, heart, kidneys, and other organs of the body. A number of biochemical, physiological, and environmental factors that increase the risk of developing arteriosclerosis have been identified and include the following:

- **High blood pressure.** This is critical in the development of atherosclerosis, which does not normally occur in the lower-pressure pulmonary arteries and veins.
- **Total cholesterol level.** This is an important risk factor, but the types of lipoproteins are even more critical. The level of LDL is the main risk factor, whereas high-density lipoprotein (HDL) seems to prevent the accumulation of cholesterol in the tissues.
- **Obesity.** This promotes other risk factors that lead to atherosclerosis.
- **Cigarette or other tobacco smoking.** This risk factor vastly increases the chances of developing atherosclerosis.
- **Diets rich in saturated fats, cholesterol, and calories.** Such diets seem to be chiefly responsible for high blood cholesterol levels and the development of atherosclerosis.
- **A family history of premature atherosclerotic disease.**
- **Diabetes.** This disease may lead to arteriosclerosis.
- **Sex.** Between the ages of 35 and 44, the death rate from coronary heart disease is 6.1 times higher among white men than that among white women. This is thought to be due to hormonal influences. Overt manifestations are rare in either sex before the age of 40 because more than a 75 percent narrowing of the arteries must occur before blood flow is seriously impeded.
- **Aging.** This process brings about degenerative arterial changes, such as dilatation and thickening and loss of elasticity.
- **Physical inactivity.** Lack of exercise increases the chances of developing complications. However, both active and inactive people may develop arteriosclerosis.
- **Type A personality characteristics.** People with such characteristics seem to be predisposed to cardiovascular disease.

Herbs for Atherosclerosis

Cardiac and vascular tonics help support the tissue of the cardiovascular system, possibly maintaining flexibility and tone in the blood vessels. Circulatory stimulants promote blood circulation and help ensure that oxygen is delivered to where it's needed. This is especially important in the face of the increased vascular resistance characteristic of atherosclerosis.

Peripheral vasodilators have obvious value because of their potential for lessening the effect of vessel blockages. Hypotensive agents are indicated to help lower elevated blood pressure, and nervines will be indicated if stress is an issue — and when isn't it! The nervines usually also act as antispasmodics. Antispasmodics help relax the muscular linings of the arteries as well as the muscles that surround the peripheral vessels.

Atherosclerosis Tincture

It's no coincidence that this prescription is similar to those used for hypertension. The causes of the different conditions, and the necessary remedies, are similar.

> 2 parts hawthorn
> 1 part linden blossom
> 1 part yarrow
> 1 part cramp bark
> 2 parts ginkgo

To make: Combine herbs and make a tincture as described on pages 113–114.

To use: Take ½ teaspoon (2.5 mL) of the tincture three times per day.

A Broader Context for Treatment

Atherosclerosis develops when genetic predispositions compound the effects of known risk factors. If you have a family history of atherosclerosis, the prudent course of action is to accept what you cannot change and change what you can. In addition to the herbal medicines described above, here are some more therapeutic recommendations:

- **Supplements.** Getting less than the recommended daily amounts of folic acid and vitamins B_6 and B_{12} may lead to elevated homocysteine levels. Homocysteine is an amino acid found normally in the body. High blood levels of homocysteine may increase the chances of developing heart disease, stroke, and circulation problems. It is thought that such elevated levels damage the arteries, predispose the blood to easy clotting, and reduce the flexibility of blood vessels. The following daily amounts of folic acid and vitamins B_6 and B_{12} are recommended for keeping homocysteine levels in check: 400 micrograms of folic acid, 2 mg of vitamin B_6, and 6 micrograms of vitamin B_{12}. Good food sources of folic acid include citrus fruits, tomatoes, vegetables, whole grains, beans, and lentils. Foods high in vitamin B_6 include meat, poultry, fish, fruits, vegetables, and grains. Major sources of vitamin B_{12} are meat, poultry, fish, and milk and other dairy products.
- **Weight.** Maintain an appropriate body weight, losing excess weight if necessary.
- **Sodium intake.** Eliminate salt from the diet.
- **Fat.** Reduce or eliminate animal fats and increase intake of vegetable oils.
- **Diet.** Eat a diet rich in fiber, complex carbohydrates, and potassium.
- **Water.** Drink at least two pints of water per day.

- **Lifestyle.** Make healthy lifestyle choices. Avoid alcohol, caffeine, and tobacco. Reduce the impact of stress.
- **Blood pressure.** Know your blood pressure. If it's high, reduce it.
- **Exercise.** Get moderate exercise — such as a 30-minute walk, swim, or bike ride—several times per week, daily if possible.
- **Relaxation.** Find a relaxation program that you enjoy, and incorporate it into your daily routine.

Dietary Supplements

A variety of nutritional supplements is essential for people with atherosclerosis. Some supplements include:

- **Magnesium:** 800 to 1200 mg per day.
- **Vitamin C:** 500 to 1000 mg three times per day.
- **Vitamin E:** 400 to 800 IU per day.
- **Flaxseed oil:** 1 tablespoon per day.
- **Coenzyme Q$_{10}$:** 50 mg two to three times per day.
- **Niacin** (in the form of inositol hexaniacinate): 500 mg three times per day with meals for 2 weeks, and then 1000 mg three times per day with meals.
- **Garlic:** the equivalent of 4000 mg of fresh garlic once per day.

CALL YOUR DOCTOR IF:

- You experience angina pain for the first time or the attacks are getting unpredictable.
- You have sudden sharp pains in the legs or feet when at rest. This may indicate a possible circulatory blockage.
- You experience unexplained problems with balance, coordination, speech, or vision. This might indicate a temporary reduction of blood to the brain.

CONGESTIVE HEART FAILURE

Congestive heart failure occurs when the heart loses some of its ability to pump blood. The loss in pumping action is usually a symptom of an underlying heart problem, such as coronary artery disease. The term *heart failure* suggests a sudden and complete stop of heart activity. Actually, the heart does not suddenly stop, but it gradually starts working less efficiently. Some people may not become aware of their condition until symptoms appear, years after the heart has started its decline. Most of the symptoms result from the congestion that develops in the lungs or from the backed-up pressure of blood in the veins of the body.

How critical the condition is depends on how much pumping capacity the heart has lost. Nearly everyone loses some pumping capacity with age. But the loss is significantly greater with heart failure, and it often results from a heart attack or other events and diseases that damage the heart. The severity of heart failure determines its effect on a person's life. The mildest form of heart failure may have little effect, but severe heart failure can interfere with even simple activities and can prove fatal.

Risk Factors

The heart loses some of its blood-pumping ability as a natural consequence of aging. However, a number of other factors can lead to a potentially life-threatening loss of pumping action. As a symptom of underlying heart disease, heart failure is closely associated with the major risk factors already discussed: smoking, high cholesterol levels, obesity, hypertension, diabetes, and abnormal blood sugar levels. Eliminating such risk factors lowers the risk of developing or aggravating heart disease and heart failure.

The presence of coronary disease is one of the greatest risk factors for heart failure. Muscle damage and scarring caused by a heart attack greatly increase the risk of heart failure. Cardiac arrhythmias, or irregular heartbeats, also raise the risk of heart failure. Any disorder that causes abnormal swelling or thickening of the heart sets the stage for heart failure.

Symptoms

Numerous symptoms are associated with heart failure, but none is specific to this condition. The symptoms include:

- **Shortness of breath.** This may result from excess fluid in the lungs. The breathing difficulties may occur at rest or during exercise. In some cases, congestion may be severe enough to prevent or interrupt sleep.
- **Fatigue.** As the heart's pumping capacity decreases, muscles and other tissues receive less oxygen and nutrition. Thus, the body cannot perform as much work, and this causes fatigue.
- **Fluid retention.** Also called *edema,* this may cause swelling of the feet; ankles; legs; and, occasionally, the abdomen.
- **Persistent coughing, especially coughing that regularly produces mucus or pink, blood-tinged sputum.** Some people develop raspy breathing or wheezing.

The Stages of Heart Failure

Heart failure usually develops slowly, and its symptoms may not appear until the condition has progressed over years. The heart naturally makes adjustments to compensate for the loss of pumping capacity. It compensates in three ways:

1. Enlargement (dilatation) allows more blood into the heart.

2. Thickening of muscle fibers (hypertrophy) strengthens the heart muscle.

3. More frequent contractions increase circulation.

By making these adjustments, the heart can temporarily make up for losses in pumping ability. However, compensation has its limits. Eventually, the heart cannot offset the lost ability to pump blood, and the signs of heart failure appear.

Herbs for Congestive Heart Failure

It would be inappropriate to explore the use of cardioactive remedies, such as foxglove, in a book of this kind. As dramatically effective as these remedies are, the key to using them safely and successfully is skilled diagnosis and interpretation by a medical doctor. Used without the necessary skills, these cardioactive plants are extremely poisonous.

The noncardioactive approach described here is effective in many situations. For example, herbs can support the work of the medication that the patient may be receiving (but they do not replace it). They can also help patients who have mild heart failure that does not warrant the use of stronger medications, especially elderly persons who have chronic congestive heart failure.

As mentioned above, cardioactive agents are the core treatment for congestive heart failure, but these are best prescribed by skilled practitioners who can carefully monitor the changes occurring in the heart and its functioning. Other types of herbal medicines that may be used to addresses heart failure include:

- Cardiac tonics, which will aid any allopathically prescribed cardiac glycosides.
- Peripheral vasodilators, which help improve circulation.
- Hypotensives, which are often appropriate because of associated hypertension.
- Diuretics, which ease water retention problems. Replacement of flushed-out potassium is essential.
- Nervines, which ease stress (that which either causes or results from the heart disease).

A Broader Perspective on Congestive Heart Failure

The dietary and lifestyle issues discussed in chapter 1 also apply to congestive heart failure:

- **Weight.** Maintain an appropriate body weight, reducing excessive weight if necessary.

Congestive Heart Failure Formula

As the primary cardioactives are out of the range of what can be safely used, our aim is to either strengthen the heart muscle or support the work of allopathically prescribed cardiac glycosides. Hawthorn, linden blossom, and garlic are essential to achieving this.

3 parts hawthorn	1 part motherwort
1 part ginkgo	1 part cramp bark
1 part linden blossom	1 part valerian
1 part dandelion leaf	

To make: Combine herbs and make a tincture as described on pages 113–114.

To use: Take ½ teaspoon (2.5 mL) of the tincture three times per day. Augment with two capsules of garlic oil taken daily with food.

- **Sodium intake.** Eliminate salt from the diet.
- **Fat.** Reduce or eliminate animal fats and increase intake of vegetable oils.
- **Diet.** Eat a diet rich in fiber, complex carbohydrates, and potassium. It should include fruits, vegetables, grains, legumes, raw nuts, and seeds.
- **Water.** Drink at least two pints of water per day.
- **Lifestyle.** Make healthy lifestyle choices. Avoid alcohol, caffeine, and tobacco. Reduce stress.
- **Blood pressure.** Know your blood pressure. If it's high, reduce it.
- **Exercise.** Get moderate exercise — such as a 30-minute walk, swim, or bicycle ride — several times per week, daily if possible.
- **Relaxation.** Find a relaxation program that you enjoy and incorporate it into your daily routine.

Dietary Supplements

A variety of supplements is essential for people with congestive heart failure. These supplements include:

- **Magnesium:** 200 to 400 mg per day.
- **Coenzyme Q$_{10}$:** 150 to 300 mg per day.
- **L-carnitine:** 300 to 500 mg three times per day.

CALL YOUR DOCTOR IF:

- You have unusual chest pain, especially if it's persistent or recurrent.
- You experience recurrent heartbeat disturbances.
- You become suddenly dizzy, light-headed, weak, or faint.

ANGINA PECTORIS

Angina pectoris, commonly known as *angina*, is a recurring pain or discomfort in the chest. It's an indication that the heart is not getting enough oxygen. It may occur when the coronary arteries, which supply blood to the heart, are obstructed and aren't letting enough blood through. Or it may occur when the heart is overworked and needs more oxygen than usual.

The main underlying cause of angina is coronary artery disease. Angina can also result from other diseases that tax the heart unduly, such as anemia, aortic valve disease, heart arrhythmias, or hyperthyroidism.

Symptoms

Angina is usually experienced as a crushing or constricting pain that starts in the center of the chest, deep behind the breastbone. The pain may radiate to other parts of the body. In some

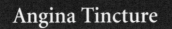

Angina Tincture

The herbal approach to angina pectoris is similar to the herbal approaches to hypertension and arteriosclerosis. Please refer to those sections for more details on the herbs used in this formula.

3 parts hawthorn   1 part linden blossom
2 parts motherwort   1 part cramp bark
1 part yarrow   1 part ginkgo

To make: Combine the herbs and make a tincture as described on page 113–114.
To use: Take ½ teaspoon (2.5 mL) of the tincture three times per day.

cases, however, the pain may be felt only in peripheral locations, such as the jaw, abdomen, or arm. The pain is sometimes confused with indigestion because both conditions cause similar tight, burning sensations. Not uncommonly, people with angina think that they're having a heart attack. The pain is similar, but angina pain doesn't last as long — it usually lasts no more than 5 minutes.

Episodes of angina occur when the heart needs more oxygen than is available from the blood nourishing the heart. Physical exertion is the most common trigger for angina. Other triggers are emotional stress, extreme cold or heat, heavy meals, alcohol, and cigarettes.

Remember, an angina attack is not a heart attack! Angina means that some of the heart muscle is temporarily not getting enough blood. The pain does not mean that the heart muscle is suffering irreversible, permanent damage.

Hawthorn for Angina Attack

You can take 1 tsp (5 mL) hawthorn tincture at the first sign of an attack. *Caution:* This should not replace the use of prescription medication.

Not all chest pain originates from the heart, and not all pain that originates from the heart is angina. For example, if the pain lasts less than 30 seconds or goes away during a deep breath, after you drink a glass of water, or after you change position, it almost certainly is not angina and isn't cause for concern. But prolonged pain that is unrelieved by rest and is accompanied by other symptoms may signal a heart attack.

Other Therapeutic Approaches for Angina

In addition to herbal medicines, other dietary and lifestyle choices may help control angina, depending on your unique life experience:

- Maintain an appropriate body weight, losing excess weight if necessary.
- Eliminate salt from the diet.
- Make healthy lifestyle choices. Avoid alcohol, caffeine, and tobacco. Reduce stress and its effects. Exercise regularly but in a way that is enjoyable to you.
- Eat a diet rich in fiber, complex carbohydrates, and potassium.
- Eat garlic and onions.
- Reduce or eliminate animal fats and increase intake of vegetable oils.

CALL YOUR DOCTOR IF:

- The attack lasts longer than 15 minutes. It could be a heart attack, and you should call 911.
- You think this may be your first angina attack.
- The attacks become more intense, frequent, prolonged, and unpredictable.
- You are taking prescription medications for angina and start to have distressing side effects.

• Supplement the diet with:
  Magnesium: 200 to 400 mg three times per day.
  Coenzyme Q$_{10}$: 150 to 300 mg per day.
  Garlic: the equivalent of 4000 mg fresh garlic, once per day.

INTERMITTENT CLAUDICATION

Peripheral vascular diseases, such as intermittent claudication, are caused by narrowing of the arteries in the legs. This narrowing restricts blood flow to muscles in the calves, thighs, and buttocks.

Symptoms

These conditions are usually symptom-free in the early stages, but the restricted availability of oxygen eventually causes major problems. The most striking symptom occurs upon exertion, such as walking. The increased need for oxygen cannot be met by the limited blood supply. This results in a buildup of lactic acid and other byproducts of enforced anaerobic metabolism in the muscles. These metabolites cause pain and cramps and restrict mobility. On resting, the pain and discomfort stop.

Herbs for Intermittent Claudication

Cardiac tonics are crucial because the immediate problem (pain in the legs) is almost certainly caused by underlying problems that affect the entire cardiovascular system. Peripheral vasodilators will facilitate the flow of blood through the extremities. Hypotensive agents will often help because there is a connection between hypertension and the development of intermittent claudication. Diuretics may be appropriate if water retention is developing. Mild remedies, such as hawthorn, may be adequate. Relaxing nervines may be indicated. Antispasmodic remedies may be appropriate in easing discomfort caused by muscular spasms.

Intermittent Claudication Formula

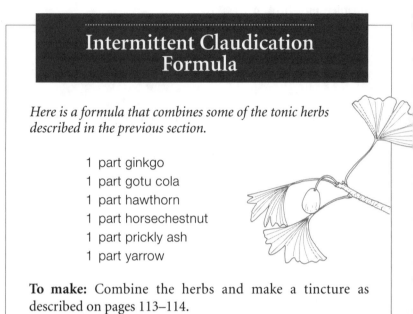

Here is a formula that combines some of the tonic herbs described in the previous section.

1 part ginkgo
1 part gotu cola
1 part hawthorn
1 part horsechestnut
1 part prickly ash
1 part yarrow

To make: Combine the herbs and make a tincture as described on pages 113–114.

To use: Take ½ teaspoon (2.5 mL) of the tincture three times per day. Supplement with 2 capsules of garlic oil taken daily with food.

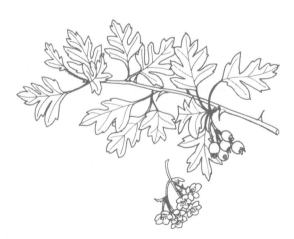

POOR CIRCULATION

Poor circulation, often experienced as coldness in the extremities (such as fingers and toes), is a common problem in cold climates.

Causes

Poor circulation has many possible causes. Thus, choosing the appropriate therapy is somewhat challenging. Herbs immediately alleviate the symptoms, but unless they also address the underlying cause or causes, no long-term change will occur. Some of the factors and body systems that may play a role in poor circulation (caused by vasodilation or vasoconstriction) include:

- The autonomic nervous system
- The endocrine system
- Basal metabolic rate
- Locally produced hormones (prostaglandins)
- Allergies
- Diet
- State of mind

It's important to note that each of these factors is, itself, multi-factorial. Consider, for example, cold hands. This could result from a whiplash injury to the neck that has led to "pinching" of the nerves that control the vascular muscles in the arms. Thus, the use of warming herbs will help relieve the symptoms but won't undo the source of the problem, which is the injured neck.

Herbs for Poor Circulation

Circulatory stimulants will promote better circulation of blood from the trunk of the body to the periphery, warming the tissue. Peripheral vasodilators also help. Vascular tonics will help the involved tissues function at maximum efficiency.

Antispasmodics ease the tightness of muscles in the limbs that might be pressing against blood vessels and reducing blood supply.

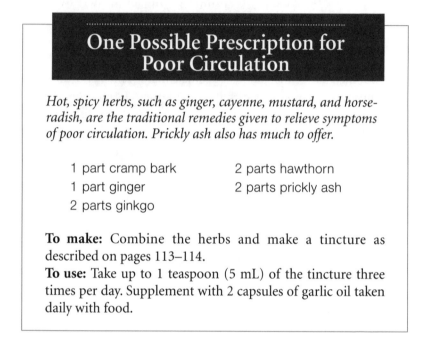

One Possible Prescription for Poor Circulation

Hot, spicy herbs, such as ginger, cayenne, mustard, and horse-radish, are the traditional remedies given to relieve symptoms of poor circulation. Prickly ash also has much to offer.

1 part cramp bark	2 parts hawthorn
1 part ginger	2 parts prickly ash
2 parts ginkgo	

To make: Combine the herbs and make a tincture as described on pages 113–114.

To use: Take up to 1 teaspoon (5 mL) of the tincture three times per day. Supplement with 2 capsules of garlic oil taken daily with food.

Other Therapeutic Approaches to Poor Circulation

In addition to herbal therapies, exercise is important to ensure that the body's metabolic rate is raised to a healthful level. Metabolic rate is a measure of the amount of work being done by the cells of the body. This rate increases during exercise. In addition, the following nutritional supplements can be very helpful:

- **Vitamin B$_3$ (nicotinic acid):** 50 mg three times per day.
- **Vitamin C:** 1000 mg once per day.
- **Vitamin E:** 600 IU once per day.
- **Evening primrose oil:** 500 mg once per day.
- **Magnesium:** 200 to 400 mg once per day.

VARICOSE VEINS

Varicose veins are a common problems, affecting between 10 and 20 percent of the U.S. population. The incidence increases with age and is most common in people over 50 years old. It is four times more common in women than in men.

A varicose vein is a superficial vessel that is abnormally twisted, lengthened, or dilated. It appears most often on the legs or thighs and causes aching and abnormal fatigue in the legs. The core problem is that some degree of reversal of blood flow occurs as a result of weak valve functioning. This causes dilation of the veins, loss of elasticity in the vein walls, and loss of tissue tone. When valves in the veins function normally, they keep blood from flowing back away from the heart. But if the efficiency of the valves decreases, some blood may stagnate in the veins, which then become swollen, twisted, and painful.

Contributing Factors

Varicose veins are a symptom of a generally poor circulatory system. Many factors may contribute, all of which can be divided into two groups.

Lack of support in the veins may be due to:
- **Heredity.** About 40 percent of people with varicose veins have a family history of varicose veins.
- **Obesity.** The fatty tissue that builds up in the legs provides inadequate support and leads to a loss of tone in the veins.
- **Age.** The aging process leads to degenerative changes in the supporting connective tissue. These changes are compounded by decreased muscular activity in older people.
- **Posture.** Occupations that involve prolonged standing or sitting increase the chances of varicose veins. This increased risk results from the pull of gravity and insufficient muscular activity in the thighs.

Increased resistance to blood flow back to the trunk may be due to:

- **Pregnancy.** While obviously not a disease, the growing baby may act as a obstacle to venous return. The condition reverses after childbirth.
- **Thrombosis.** Blood clots may form blockages in the blood vessels.
- **Tumors.** Uterine fibroids, to name one example, may become obstructive.
- **Fashion.** Constriction caused by tight clothing around the legs and waist will weaken the tissue.

Herbs for Varicose Veins

Vascular tonics (such as hawthorn, horsechestnut, and yarrow) will help the tissues regain tone and strength. Bioflavonoid-rich and flavonoid-rich herbs such as horsechestnut are especially useful, although they usually don't work quickly. Circulatory stimulants such as prickly ash and ginkgo help improve the flow of blood back into the trunk of the body. Astringents such as yarrow and witch hazel can be applied externally to help the work of the vascular tonics. Anti-inflammatories such as horsechestnut will ease the localized inflammation and discomfort. When used externally, emollients or demulcents such as comfrey will lessen localized discomfort.

Other Therapeutic Approaches for Varicose Veins

Lifestyle factors are very important in the long-term treatment of this sometimes intransigent condition. Diet is as important for this condition as it is for the rest of the cardiovascular system. Guidelines similar to those for the disorders already described apply for varicosity.

Varicose Vein Formula

In Europe, horsechestnut has traditionally been considered an effective remedy specifically for varicose veins.

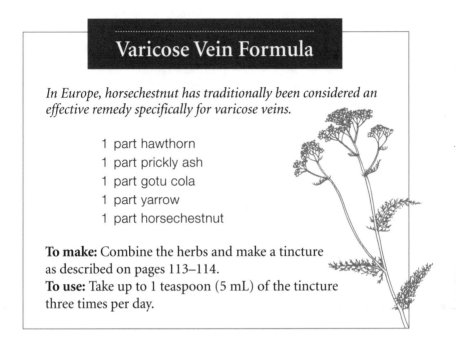

   1 part hawthorn
   1 part prickly ash
   1 part gotu cola
   1 part yarrow
   1 part horsechestnut

To make: Combine the herbs and make a tincture as described on pages 113–114.
To use: Take up to 1 teaspoon (5 mL) of the tincture three times per day.

Varicose Vein Lotion

This lotion may be applied to legs and thighs to ease irritation and discomfort.

   5 tbs (80 mL) distilled witch hazel
   2 tsp (10 mL) horsechestnut tincture
   2 tsp (10 mL) comfrey tincture
   Rose water (optional, for fragrance)

To make: Combine all ingredients in a jar.
To use: Apply externally in liberal amounts as needed.

Physical Changes

The key factor in alleviating varicose veins is avoiding postures or situations that make it difficult for blood in the legs to return to the circulation. Anything that counteracts the effects of gravity will be helpful. For example:

- **Resting with the legs higher than the head for at least 10 minutes every day.** This may be done through the inverted postures of yoga, by using a slant-board, or simply by lying on the floor with your legs and feet supported by a chair. The foot of the bed can be elevated 6 to 12 inches to facilitate drainage at night.
- **Gentle exercise.** Walking and gentle stretching exercises are suitable, but jogging, skipping, aerobics, and other exercises that involve repeated impact can do more harm than good.
- **Aromatherapy.** When used in a broad holistic context, this can help improve the general tone of the veins. Cypress oil has a good reputation for strengthening the veins in the legs. It can be used as a bath oil or can be applied very gently over the area of the affected veins.
- **Massage.** This can be used above the affected area of the vein, but it must never be used below the varicosity because doing so will increase pressure in the vein.

Diet and Supplements

You can make many dietary changes to help reduce the likelihood of developing varicose veins. Recommended changes include:

- Maintaining an appropriate body weight and losing excess weight if necessary.
- Eliminating salt from the diet.
- Avoiding alcohol, caffeine, and tobacco.

- Eating a diet rich in fiber, complex carbohydrates, and potassium.

In addition, the following nutritional supplements can be very helpful:

- Vitamin A: 10,000 IU per day.
- Vitamin B complex: 10 to 100 mg per day.
- Vitamin C with bioflavonoids: 1000 to 3000 mg per day.
- Vitamin E: 200 to 600 IU per day.
- Magnesium: 800 to 1200 mg per day.
- Zinc: 15 to 30 mg per day.

A GUIDE TO
THE HEALING HERBS

This chapter offers more in-depth information on the herbs mentioned in the previous chapters of this book. Most of these herbs are available at good natural food stores or through mail-order suppliers of high-quality herbs.

❋ARNICA (*Arnica montana*, L. Asteraceae)

Part Used: Flower heads.
Actions: Anti-inflammatory, vulnerary.
Indications: This herb is toxic and should not be taken internally (however, the homeopathic preparation is entirely safe to take internally). It is one of the best remedies for external local healing. It helps relieve rheumatic pain as well as the inflammation and pain of phlebitis and similar conditions. Phlebitis is an inflammation of a vein, often accompanied by a blood clot, or thrombus, in the affected vein. When a blood clot is present, the condition is known as *thrombophlebitis*. Blood clot formation may follow injury, surgery, childbirth, or prolonged bed rest or may be associated with infection. The chief danger is that the clot may dislodge and travel to a vital organ, causing serious damage.
Preparation and Dosage: You can prepare your own tincture of arnica by pouring 1 pint (½ L) 70 percent alcohol over 2 ounces

(50 g) freshly picked flowers. Place in a clear glass container, seal tightly, and let stand for at least a week in the sun or in a warm place. Filter the tincture, then use as needed. To store, put the tincture in a sealed container and keep it out of direct sunlight. The tincture, or a cream containing the tincture, should be applied topically to reduce the pain and discomfort of bruising or local inflammation.

> ## CAUTION!
>
> Arnica is toxic and should not be taken internally. Death can result from even low internal doses.

BUGLEWEED (*Lycopus europaeus*, L. Lamiaceae)

Parts Used: Aerial parts.

Actions: Diuretic, peripheral vasoconstrictor, astringent, nervine, antitussive.

Indications: Bugleweed may be used for overactive thyroid glands, especially when symptoms include difficulty breathing, palpitation, and shaking. It is also helpful for a weak heart and the corresponding buildup of water in the body. As a sedative, it helps ease irritating coughs, especially those of a nervous origin.

Preparation and Dosage: To make an infusion, pour 1 cup boiling water over 1 teaspoon (5 mL) dried herb; let infuse 10–15 minutes. Drink 3 times per day.

When using a tincture, take 1–2 mL (¼ tsp) 3 times per day.

CAYENNE (*Capsicum frutescens*, L. Solanaceae)

Part Used: Fruit.

Actions: Stimulant, carminative, anticatarrhal, sialagogue, rubefacient, antimicrobial.

Indications: Cayenne is the most useful of the systemic stimulants specifically for the circulatory system. It stimulates blood flow by strengthening the heart, arteries, capillaries, and nerves. A general tonic, it is also helpful for both the circulatory and digestive systems. It may be used for flatulent dyspepsia and colic and may help relieve insufficient peripheral circulation that leads to cold hands and feet and possibly chilblains. When applied externally, it is a local circulation stimulant for problems such as lumbago and rheumatic pains. As an ointment used in moderation, cayenne helps unbroken chilblains. As a gargle for laryngitis, it combines well with myrrh. This combination is also a good antiseptic wash.

Preparation and Dosage: To make an infusion, pour 1 cup boiling water over ½–1 teaspoon (2.5–5 mL) dried herb powder; infuse 10 minutes. Mix 1 tablespoon (15 mL) infusion with hot water and drink as needed.

CLEAVERS (*Galium aparine*, L. Rubiaceae)

Actions: Diuretic, anti-inflammatory, tonic, astringent.

Indications: Cleavers is a valuable plant; it may be the best tonic for the lymphatic system and can be used safely for a wide range of problems involving this system. These include swollen glands (lymphadenitis) anywhere in the body, especially in tonsillitis and adenoid trouble. Cleavers is helpful in skin conditions, especially those that cause dry or scaly skin, such as psoriasis. It can be used to treat cystitis and other painful urinary conditions, and it may be combined with urinary demulcents. Cleavers has long been used to treat ulcers and tumors, probably because it causes lymphatic drainage, which helps detoxify tissue.

Preparation and Dosage: To make an infusion, pour 1 cup boiling water over 2–3 teaspoons (5–7.5 mL) dried herb; infuse 10–15 minutes. Drink 3 times per day.

When using a tincture, take 4–8 mL 3 times per day.

COLEUS (*Coleus forskohlii*, Lamiaceae)

Part Used: Root.

Actions: Hypotensive, cardiotonic, vasodilating, antispasmodic.

Indications: The core effects of coleus result from the action of a constituent called *forskolin.* This substance activates an enzyme known as *adenylate cyclase,* which increases cellular levels of cyclic adenosine monophosphate. This process leads to an array of pharmacologic responses in various tissues of the body, ranging from reduction of elevated blood pressure and relaxation of smooth muscle to dilatation of the bronchioles in the lungs and reduction of pressure within the eye. Coleus is an important heart and circulatory tonic that is used to treat congestive heart failure and poor coronary blood flow.

Preparation and Dosage: To make a decoction, pour 1 cup boiling water over 2–5 g root and simmer 10–15 minutes. Drink 3 times per day.

Standardized extracts should contain 18 percent forskolin. Take 50 mg 2 to 3 times per day.

CORN (*Zea mays,* L. Poaceae)

Part Used: Silk.

Actions: Diuretic, demulcent, anti-inflammatory, tonic.

Indications: As a soothing diuretic, corn silk is helpful for any irritation of the urinary system. It is used for renal problems in children and, when combined with other herbs, serves as a urinary demulcent in the treatment of cystitis, urethritis, prostatitis, and the like.

Combinations: Take with couchgrass, bearberry, buchu, or yarrow for the treatment of cystitis.

Preparation and Dosage: To make an infusion, pour 1 cup boiling water over 2 teaspoons (5 mL) dried herb; infuse 10–15 minutes. Drink 3 times per day.

When using a tincture, take 3–6 mL 3 times per day.

⊕COUCHGRASS (*Elytrigia repens* ssp. *repens*, [L.] Beauvois, Poaceae)

Part Used: Rhizome.

Actions: Diuretic, demulcent, antimicrobial.

Indications: Couchgrass (often called quackgrass in North America) may be used for urinary infections, such as cystitis, urethritis, and prostatitis. Its demulcent properties soothe irritation and inflammation. It is valuable for the treatment of enlarged prostate glands. It may also be used for kidney stones and gravel. As a tonic diuretic, couchgrass has been used with other herbs in the treatment of rheumatism.

Combinations: For urinary tract infections, couchgrass may be used with bearberry, buchu, or yarrow. It can be combined with hydrangea for prostate problems.

Preparation and Dosage: To make a decoction, put 2 teaspoons (10 mL) cut rhizome in 1 cup water, bring to boil, and let simmer 10 minutes. Drink 3 times per day.

When using a tincture, take 2–4 mL 3 times per day.

⊕CRAMP BARK (*Viburnum opulus*, L. Caprifoliaceae)

Part Used: Dried bark.

Actions: Antispasmodic, anti-inflammatory, nervine, hypotensive, astringent, emmenagogue.

Indications: This herb has a richly deserved reputation as a relaxer of muscular tension and spasm. It has two main uses: for muscular cramps and for ovarian and uterine muscle problems. Cramp bark relaxes the uterus and thus relieves painful cramps associated with menstrual periods (dysmenorrhea). In a similar way, it may be used to protect against miscarriage. Its astringent action gives it a role in the treatment of excessive blood loss during menstruation and for bleeding associated with menopause.

Preparation and Dosage: To make a decoction, put 2 teaspoons (10 mL) dried herb into 1 cup water. Bring to a boil and simmer gently 10–15 minutes. Drink hot 3 times per day.

When using a tincture, take 4–8 mL 3 times per day.

DANDELION (*Taraxacum officinale,* Asteraceae)

Part Used: Root or leaf.

Actions: Diuretic, hepatic, cholagogue, antirheumatic, laxative, tonic, bitter.

Indications: Dandelion leaf is a powerful diuretic, and its effects are similar to those of the drug furosemide. Unlike this drug, however, which can cause a loss of vital potassium from the body, dandelion is one of the best natural sources of potassium. It's an ideally balanced diuretic that may be used safely for water retention due to heart problems. Dandelion root may also be used to relieve inflammation and congestion of the liver and gall bladder. It is specifically indicated in cases of congestive jaundice. As part of a wider treatment for muscular rheumatism, it can be very effective. This herb is a valuable general tonic and may be the best widely applicable diuretic and liver tonic.

Combinations: For liver and gallbladder problems, dandelion may be used with balmony or barberry. For water retention, it may be used with couchgrass or yarrow.

Preparation and Dosage: To make a decoction, put 2–3 teaspoons (10–15 mL) root into 1 cup water, bring to boil, and gently simmer 10–15 minutes. Drink 3 times per day.

When using a tincture, take 1–2 teaspoons (5–10 mL) 3 times per day.

The leaves may be eaten raw in salads.

FEVERFEW (*Chrysanthemum parthenium,* (L.) Bernh. Asteraceae)

Part Used: Leaves.

Actions: Anti-inflammatory, vasodilator, bitter, emmenagogue.

Indications: Feverfew has regained its deserved reputation as a primary remedy for the treatment of migraine headaches, especially those that are relieved by applying warmth to the head. Feverfew may also help arthritis during the painful inflammatory stage. Dizziness and tinnitus may be eased, especially when feverfew is used with other remedies. Feverfew relieves painful menstrual periods and sluggish menstrual flow.

Feverfew is the only herb used in European herbalism that is known to be specific for the treatment of migraine. It is also the best example of a remedy well-known to medical herbalists that has recently been accepted and used by allopathic medicine. It has been used throughout recorded medical history as a bitter tonic and remedy for severe headaches. Through wide media coverage in recent years, the herb has gained a well-deserved reputation as a "cure" for migraine. Clinicians at the London Migraine Clinic observed that patients were reporting marked improvements when they took the herb. Thankfully, these doctors had the inquiring and open minds of the true scientist and so started their own investigations into the claims for feverfew.

Long-term users often report beneficial side effects of feverfew use, such as relief from depression, nausea, and arthritic pain. The herb seems to inhibit secretion of the granular contents from platelets and neutrophils in the blood. This may be relevant to the therapeutic value of feverfew in migraine and other conditions, such as osteoarthritis. Pharmacologists say it is very likely that the sesquiterpene

CAUTION!

Feverfew should not be used during pregnancy because of its stimulant action on the uterus. In addition, the fresh leaves may cause mouth ulcers in sensitive people.

lactones inhibit prostaglandins and histamine released during the inflammatory process, thus preventing spasms of the blood vessels in the head that trigger migraine attacks. As with all such impressive research findings, do not lose sight of the importance of whole plant activity rather than simply "active" ingredients.

Preparation and Dosage: It is best to use the equivalent of one fresh leaf, 1–3 times per day. Tinctures or tablets are also adequate. When using freeze-dried leaf preparations, take 50–100 mg per day.

FIGWORT (*Scrophularia nodosa*, Juss. Scrophularaceae)

Part Used: Aerial parts.
Actions: Alterative, diuretic, laxative, heart stimulant.
Indications: Figwort is mainly used for the treatment of skin problems. It acts in a broad way to help the body function well, bringing about a state of inner cleanliness. It may be used for eczema, psoriasis, and any skin condition accompanied by itching and irritation. Part of figwort's cleansing ability stems from its purgative and diuretic actions. Figwort may be used as a mild laxative in constipation. Since it is a heart stimulant, figwort should be avoided where there is any abnormally rapid heartbeat (tachycardia).

Preparation and Dosage: To make an infusion, pour 1 cup boiling water over 1–3 teaspoons (5–15 mL) dried leaves; infuse 10–15 minutes. Drink 3 times per day.

When using a tincture, take 2–4 mL 3 times per day.

> **CAUTION!**
>
> Figwort should not be used by people with abnormally rapid heartbeat (tachycardia).

GARLIC (*Allium sativum*, L. Liliaceae)

Part Used: Bulb.
Actions: Antimicrobial, diaphoretic, cholagogue, hypotensive, antispasmodic.
Indications: Garlic has an international reputation for lowering

elevated blood pressure and blood cholesterol and for improving the health of the cardiovascular system. Garlic should be considered a basic food that will augment the body's health and protect it in general.

Garlic aids and supports the body in ways that no other herb does. It is one of the most effective antimicrobial plants available, acting on bacteria, viruses, and alimentary parasites. The volatile oil is an effective agent that is largely secreted via the lungs. Thus, the oil is effective for treating chronic bronchitis, respiratory catarrh, and recurrent colds and influenza. Garlic may be helpful in the treatment of whooping cough and, as part of a broader approach, bronchitic asthma. In general, garlic may be used to prevent most infectious conditions, digestive as well as respiratory. It's especially good for digestive problems because it supports the development of the natural bacterial flora while killing pathogenic organisms.

Combinations: For microbial infections, garlic combines well with echinacea.

Preparation and Dosage: Eat 1 clove fresh garlic 3 times per day. If the smell becomes a problem, take 2–3 garlic oil capsules per day as a preventive measure; increase to 3 times per day when an infection occurs.

GENTIAN (*Gentiana lutea*, L. Gentianaceae)

Part Used: Dried root.

Actions: Bitter, sialagogue, hepatic, cholagogue, antimicrobial, anthelmintic, emmenagogue.

Indications: Gentian is an excellent bitter that stimulates the appetite and digestion. It promotes the production of saliva, gastric juices, and bile. It also accelerates emptying of the stomach. It is indicated for lack of appetite, sluggishness of the digestive system, dyspepsia, and flatulence. Through the stimulation of digestion, it has a generally fortifying effect.

Preparation and Dosage: To make a decoction, put ½ teaspoon (2.5 mL) shredded root in 1 cup water and boil 5 minutes. Drink warm 15–30 minutes before meals or as needed.

When using a tincture, take 1–2 mL 3 times per day or as needed.

GERMAN CHAMOMILE (*Matricaria recutita*, L. Asteraceae)

Part Used: Flowering tops.
Actions: Nervine, antispasmodic, carminative, anti-inflammatory, antimicrobial, bitter, vulnerary.
Indications: A comprehensive list of the medical uses of chamomile would be long. Some of the conditions for which chamomile is used are insomnia, anxiety, menopausal depression, loss of appetite, dyspepsia, diarrhea, colic, flu symptoms, migraine, neuralgia, teething, vertigo, motion sickness, conjunctivitis, inflamed skin, and urticaria.

Chamomile is probably the most widely used relaxing nervine herb in the western world. It relaxes and tones the nervous system and is especially valuable when anxiety and tension produce digestive symptoms such as gas, colic pains, or even ulcers. It makes a wonderful late-night tea to ensure restful sleep. It can also be added to bath water to help soothe anxious children or teething infants.

As an antispasmodic herb, chamomile works on the peripheral nerves and muscles and thus indirectly relaxes the whole body. When the physical body is relaxed, ease in the mind and heart follows. Chamomile can prevent or ease cramps in the muscles, including those in the legs and abdomen.

Chamomile is rich in essential oil and acts on the digestive system, promoting proper function. This usually involves soothing the walls of the intestines, easing griping pains, and helping remove gas.

Chamomile is a mild antimicrobial, helping the body destroy or resist pathogenic microorganisms. As an anticatarrhal, it helps the body remove excess mucus buildup in the sinus area. It may be used for head colds and allergic reactions, such as hay fever.

Preparation and Dosage: To make an infusion, pour 1 cup boiling water over 2–3 tablespoons (30–45 mL) dried herb; infuse 10 minutes. Take 3–4 times per day.

When using a tincture, take 1–4 mL 3 times per day.

GINGER (*Zingiber officinale,* Roscoe Zingiberaceae)

Part Used: Rhizome.

Actions: Stimulant, carminative, antispasmodic, rubefacient, diaphoretic, emmenagogue.

Indications: Ginger may be used as a stimulant of the peripheral circulation for impaired circulation, chilblains, and cramps. In feverish conditions, it acts as a useful diaphoretic, promoting perspiration. As a gargle, it may relieve sore throats. Externally, it is the base of many fibrositis and muscle-sprain treatments. Ginger has also been used worldwide as an aromatic carminative and pungent appetite stimulant. In India and other countries with hot and humid climates, ginger is eaten daily and is a well-known remedy for digestive problems. Its widespread use is the result not only of its flavor but also its antioxidant and antimicrobial effects.

Preparation and Dosage: To make an infusion, pour 1 cup boiling water over l teaspoon (5 mL) fresh root (grated or chopped); infuse 5 minutes. Drink as needed.

CAUTION!

Do not use ginger during pregnancy or breastfeeding.

People with gallstones should consult a medical professional before using ginger.

Do not use ginger if you are taking an antibiotic medication, because ginger may mask symptoms of toxicity from this medication.

To make a decoction using dried root in powdered or finely chopped form, add 1½ teaspoons (7.5 mL) to 1 cup water. Bring to boil and simmer 5–10 minutes. Drink as needed.

GINKGO (*Ginkgo biloba*, L. Ginkgoaceae)

Part Used: Leaves. In oriental herbalism, the seed kernel is used extensively.

Actions: Anti-inflammatory, vasodilatory, relaxant, digestive bitter, uterine stimulant.

Indications: Traditionally known as an antimicrobial and antitubercular agent, ginkgo has recently been shown to also affect brain function and cerebral circulation. Clinically, it is proving effective for a range of vascular disorders. Its use has been suggested for vertigo, tinnitus, inner-ear disturbances, memory and mental impairment, anxiety, dementia, Alzheimer's disease, complications of stroke, diminished sight and hearing due to vascular insufficiency, intermittent claudication, Raynaud's phenomenon, and many more conditions.

Preparation and Dosage: Ginkgo is becoming available in many different forms. The clinically recommended dose is 40 mg dried herb 3 times per day.

When ginkgo is used for organic brain disorders, the German E Commission (the German equivalent of the U.S. Food and Drug Administration) recommends taking 120–240 mg native dry extract in two or three doses. When gingko is used for cardiovascular problems elsewhere in the body, the Commission recommends 120–160 mg in two to three doses.

HAWTHORN (*Crataegus laevigata* and *C. monogyna*, L. Rosaceae)

Part Used: Flowers, leaves, berries.

Actions: Cardiotonic, diuretic, astringent, hypotensive.

Indications: Hawthorn can be considered a specific remedy for most cardiovascular diseases. It is a tonic in the true sense. The therapeutic benefits are gained only when the whole plant preparation is used. When the isolated constituents were tested separately in the laboratory, their individual effects were insignificant. Another example of herbal synergy!

Hawthorn may be used to treat cardiovascular degenerative diseases, including myocardial problems and coronary artery disease. The herb eases and helps prevent angina pectoris and similar symptoms. Hawthorn may also be helpful for people who do not have disease but have lost some cardiac function because of old age. The herb is nontoxic and may be appropriate for long-term use.

Other uses include postinfarction recovery, essential hypertension (used in conjunction with hypotensives), heart weakness after infectious diseases, and cardiac arrhythmias.

Dosage and Preparation: As a tonic, use 2 teaspoons dried berries in an infusion to be drunk three times a day. As part of treatment for cardiovascular problems, take ½ teaspoon of the tincture three times a day.

Hawthorn Berry Conserve

Hawthorn need not be seen as a "medicine" but can be considered a food. An example of how it can be used as a heart tonic every day is this tasty conserve, which can be spread on bread, crackers, or fruit.

1. Place a large handful of dried hawthorn berries in a bowl and add apple juice to cover the tops of berries by 2 inches. Add a cinnamon stick.
2. Place in refrigerator and allow to soak overnight.
3. Remove cinnamon stick and sweeten the soaked berries with a little honey.

⊕Horsechestnut (*Aesculus hippocastanum*, L. Hippocastanaceae)

Part Used: Fruit, seeds, pericarp (walls of the fruit).

Actions: Astringent, anti-inflammatory.

Indications: The unique actions of horsechestnut affect the vessels of the circulatory system. Horsechestnut seems to increase the strength and tone of the veins in particular. It may be used internally to help treat phlebitis, inflammation in the veins, varicosity, and hemorrhoids. Externally, it may be used as a lotion for the same conditions and for leg ulcers.

Combinations: Horsechestnut may be used with other cardiovascular tonics, such as hawthorn, linden, ginkgo, and yarrow.

Preparation and Dosage: To make an infusion, pour 1 cup boiling water over 1–2 teaspoons (5–10 mL) dried herb; infuse 10–15 minutes. Drink 3 times per day or use as an external lotion.

When using a tincture, take 1–4 mL 3 times per day.

> # CAUTION!
>
> Do not confuse horsechestnut with its North American relative *Aesculus glabra,* known by the common name *buckeye.*

⊕Kava Kava (*Piper methysticum,* G. Forst. Piperaceae)

Part Used: Rhizome.

Actions: Relaxing nervine, hypnotic, antispasmodic, local anesthetic, antifungal.

Indications: Kava kava is a safe treatment for anxiety that, when used at normal therapeutic doses, does not dampen alertness. In one double-blind, placebo-controlled study, 29 subjects were treated with 100 mg of kava extract (standardized to contain 70 percent kava lactones) three times a day for four weeks. Compared to the placebo group, the kava group experienced significant decreases in symptoms of anxiety, as measured on the Hamilton

Anxiety Scale (Kinzler *et al. Arzeneimittelforschung,* 1991;41:584–588). Another study found kava kava to be effective for decreasing anxiety associated with menopause (Volz and Kieser. *Pharmacopsychiatry,* 1997;30:1–5).

The herb compares favorably to prescription medications such as benzodiazepines, which are often used to treat anxiety disorders. It does not impair reaction time and seems to improve concentration. It possesses a mild antidepressant activity, and this makes it suitable for the treatment of anxiety associated with minor forms of depression.

Kava kava is an effective muscle relaxant and is therefore useful for the treatment of conditions associated with skeletal muscle spasm and tension, such as headaches due to neck tension. It is also helpful for mild insomnia. Its local anesthetic action on mucous membranes makes kava kava useful for pain control in oral conditions. Kavain possesses significant analgesic effects in animal studies, apparently via nonopiate pathways (Jamieson and Duffield. *Clin Exp Pharmacol Physiol,* 1990;17:495–507). Subcutaneous injections have been known to provide anesthesia for several hours to several days. Kava is a very useful muscle relaxant, antispasmodic for conditions of the cardiovascular system such as hypertension.

A side effect of heavy kava kava consumption is a skin rash known as kava dermopathy. This is typically seen only in people who consume large amounts of kava beverages over the long term, as is common in Polynesia. However, dosages of 300–800 mg per day have been known to cause the rash (Keller and Klohs. *Lloydia,* 1963; 26:1–15).

Preparation and Dosage: The recommended dose depends on the concentration of kava lactones. Generally, this is approximately 100 mg of the 70 percent standardized extract. In a 30 percent concentration, the dosage would be about 200 mg 3 times per day.

CAUTION!

Do not use kava kava during pregnancy or breastfeeding. People with depression should consult a medical professional before using kava kava.

KOLA (*Cola acuminata,* [Beauv.] Schott & Endl., Sterculiaceae)

Part Used: Seed.

Actions: Stimulant to central nervous system, antidepressive, astringent, diuretic.

Indications: Kola has a marked stimulating effect on human consciousness. It can be used whenever direct stimulation is needed, which is less often than is usually thought. In the short term, kola may be used to relieve nervous debility in states of atony and weakness. It can act as a specific treatment for nervous diarrhea. It may be helpful in states of depression and for relieving some varieties of migraine.

Preparation and Dosage: To make a decoction, put 1–2 teaspoons (5–10 mL) powdered nuts in 1 cup water, bring to a boil, and simmer gently 10–15 minutes. Drink as needed.

When using a tincture, take 1–2 mL 3 times per day.

LAVENDER (*Lavandula angustifolia,* Miller, Lamiaceae)

Part Used: Flowers.

Actions: Carminative, antispasmodic, antidepressant, rubefacient, emmenagogue, hypotensive.

Indications: This beautiful herb has many uses: culinary, cosmetic, and medicinal. It is beneficial for headaches, especially those related to stress. Lavender can be effective in clearing depression, especially if used with other remedies. As a gentle, strengthening tonic of the nervous system, it may be used in states of nervous debility and exhaustion. It can be used to soothe and promote natural sleep. Externally, the oil can serve as a stimulating liniment to help ease the aches and pains of rheumatism.

Preparation and Dosage: To make an infusion, pour 1 cup boiling water over 1 teaspoon (5 mL) dried herb; infuse 10 minutes. Drink 3 times per day.

For external use, the essential oil can be inhaled, rubbed on the skin, or used in baths.

LILY OF THE VALLEY (*Convallaria majalis,* Liliaceae)

Part Used: Leaves and flowers.
Actions: Cardioactive, diuretic.
Indications: Lily of the valley is used by European herbalists as an alternative to foxglove. Both herbs have a profound effect in heart failure, whether this condition is due to cardiovascular problems or to chronic lung problems, such as emphysema. Lily of the valley encourages the heart to beat more slowly, regularly, and efficiently. It is also strongly diuretic, reducing blood volume and lowering blood pressure. It is better tolerated than foxglove because it does not accumulate in the body to the same degree. Relatively low doses are required to support heart rate and rhythm and to increase urine production.

> # CAUTION!
>
> Use lily of the valley only only if you are under professional supervision.

LINDEN (*Tilia* species, Tiliaceae)

Part Used: Dried flowers.
Actions: Nervine, antispasmodic, hypotensive, diaphoretic, diuretic, anti-inflammatory, emmenagogue, astringent.
Indications: Linden is a relaxing remedy for use in nervous tension. It has a reputation as a prophylactic against arteriosclerosis and hypertension. It is considered uniquely relevant for the treating raised blood pressure associated with arteriosclerosis and nervous tension. Because of its relaxing action combined with a general effect on the circulatory system, it has a role in treating some forms of migraine. Its diaphoretic actions and its relaxing effects explain its value in feverish colds and flu.
Preparation and Dosage: To make an infusion, pour 1 cup boiling water over 1 teaspoon (5 mL) blossoms; infuse 10 minutes. Drink 3 times per day. For a diaphoretic effect in people with fever, use 2–3 teaspoons (10–15 mL).

When using a tincture, take 1–2 mL 3 times per day.

LOBELIA (*Lobelia inflata*, L. Campanulaceae)

Part Used: Aerial parts.

Actions: Antiasthmatic, antispasmodic, expectorant, emetic, nervine.

Indications: Lobelia is one of the most useful systemic relaxants available. It has a general depressant action on the central and autonomic nervous system and on neuromuscular action. It may be used to treat many conditions and is often combined with other herbs to further their effectiveness when relaxation is needed. Lobelia's primary specific use is for bronchitic asthma and bronchitis. An analysis of the action of the alkaloids present — lobeline and isolobelanine — reveals apparently paradoxical effects. Lobeline is a powerful respiratory stimulant, while isolobelanine is an emetic and respiratory relaxant. Lobelia stimulates catarrhal secretion and expectoration while relaxing the muscles of the respiratory system. The overall action is a truly holistic combination of stimulation and relaxation.

Preparation and Dosage: To make an infusion, pour 1 cup boiling water over ¼ to ½ teaspoons (1.75–2.5 mL) dried leaves; allow to infuse 10–15 minutes. Drink 3 times per day.

When using a tincture, take ½ mL 3 times per day.

> # CAUTION!
>
> Do not use lobelia during pregnancy. May cause nausea and vomiting. Use dried herb only.

MA HUANG (*Ephedra sinica*, Staph. Ephedraceae)

Part Used: Aerial stems.

Actions: Vasodilator, hypertensive, circulatory stimulant, antiallergic.

Indications: Ma huang has been used in China for at least 5000 years to treat a range of health problems, especially those of the respiratory system. This ancient medicinal plant was also mentioned in the Hindu Vedas (ancient holy writings). With the discovery of the alkaloids in ma huang, traditional herbal wisdom has been verified, providing modern medicine with important healing tools.

A Note on Ma Huang's Side Effects

A range of therapeutically active alkaloids are found in ma huang, and they sometimes amount to 2 percent of the dried herb. The alkaloids were first isolated in 1887 and came into extensive use in the 1930s. Various species of Asian *Ephedra* are sources of the widely used alkaloids ephedrine and pseudoephedrine, mainly *Ephedra sinica* and *E. equisetina* from China and *E. gerardiana* from India.

The alkaloids present in ephedra have apparently opposite effects on the body. The overall action, however, is one of balance and benefit. A brief review of the pharmacology of these alkaloids might be illuminating. Ephedrine was the first ma huang alkaloid to find wide use in western medicine, being hailed as a "cure" for asthma because of its ability to relax the airways in the lungs. Unfortunately, as often happens with "miracle cures," it soon became clear that this isolated constituent of *Ephedra* had unacceptable side effects that dramatically limited its use: Specifically, ephedrine stimulated the autonomic nervous system, causing elevated blood pressure.

When researchers studied the whole plant, only a slight blood pressure elevation was found. This led to the discovery that pseudoephedrine, another of the alkaloids present, slightly reduces both heart rate and blood pressure, avoiding the side effects that often accompany use of ephedrine. Pseudoephedrine is an effective bronchodilator. Although equivalent in strength to ephedrine, pseudoephedrine causes less stimulation of the nervous system, thus resulting in less vasoconstriction, tachycardia (heart palpitations), and other cardiovascular symptoms.

Clinical studies have found insignificant side effects with pseudoephedrine. The efficacy and safety of pseudoephedrine are recognized by the U.S. Food and Drug Administration, which has approved its use in over-the-counter medications as a safe and effective nasal decongestant. The naturally occurring alkaloids have been synthesized in the laboratory, however, even though they have the same molecular structure, they have different physical properties. The natural form rotates polarized light to the left, while the synthetic form is optically inactive. In practice, the natural form is tolerated better and has less effect on the heart.

All of these studies confirm that the traditional uses for *Ephedra sinica* are effective and safe for nasal congestion and sinus pressure, whether these problems are due to the common cold, allergies, or sinusitis. The herb is used with great success for asthma and associated conditions because of its power to relieve spasms in the bronchial tubes. It is thus used to treat bronchial asthma, bronchitis, and whooping cough. It also reduces allergic reactions and thus has a role in the treatment of hay fever and other allergies. It may be used for treating low blood pressure and circulatory insufficiency.

Preparation and Dosage: To make a decoction, put 1–2 teaspoons dried herb in 1 cup water. Bring to a boil and simmer 10–15 minutes. Drink 3 times per day.

When using a tincture, take 1–4 mL 3 times per day.

CAUTION!

Ma huang should not be used by people with cardiovascular conditions, thyroid disease, anxiety disorders, glaucoma, depression, or diabetes. Not for use by men who have difficulty urinating because of prostate enlargement. Should not be taken with other central nervous system stimulants or MAO inhibitors.

MILK THISTLE (*Silybum marianum*, [L.] Gaertn. Asteraceae)

Part Used: Seeds.
Actions: Hepatic, galactogogue, demulcent, cholagogue.
Indications: Milk thistle can be used to increase the secretion and flow of bile from the liver and gallbladder. Its traditional use as a liver tonic has been supported by research showing that it contains constituents that protect liver cells from chemical damage. It is used for a range of liver and gallbladder conditions, including hepatitis and cirrhosis. Historically, this herb has been used in Europe as a liver tonic. It may also have value in the treatment of chronic uterine problems.

Many of the chemical components in milk thistle herb have been shown to protect liver cells. These components are all flavones and flavolignins, the best-studied of which is silymarin. Silymarin reverses the effects of highly toxic alkaloids, such as phalloidin and amanitin from the "avenging angel" mushroom (*Amanita phalloides*). The pharmacodynamics, site, and mechanism of action of silymarin are becoming well understood, giving insights into the metabolic basis of this herb's activity. As its name implies, milk thistle promotes milk secretion and is perfectly safe for breast-feeding mothers.

Preparation and Dosage: To make an infusion, pour 1 cup boiling water over 1 teaspoon (5 mL) ground seeds; infuse 10–15 minutes. Drink 3 times per day.

MOTHERWORT (*Leonurus cardiaca*, L. Lamiaceae)

Part Used: Aerial parts.
Actions: Nervine, emmenagogue, antispasmodic, hepatic, cardiac tonic, hypotensive.
Indications: The many names of this plant show its range of uses. *Motherwort* hints at its relevance to menstrual and uterine conditions, while *cardiaca* (the species name) indicates its usefulness in heart and circulation treatments. It is valuable in the stimulation

of delayed or suppressed menstruation, especially when anxiety or tension is involved. It is also a useful relaxing tonic for aiding menopausal changes. It may be used to ease false labor pains. It is an excellent tonic for the heart, strengthening without straining. It is considered to be a specific treatment in cases of tachycardia (heart palpitations), especially those caused by anxiety. It may be used for all heart conditions that are associated with anxiety and tension. Chinese research mentioned in *Potters New Cyclopedia of Botanical Drugs and Preparations* found that motherwort reduced blood platelet aggregation and decreased levels of blood lipids.

Preparation and Dosage: To make an infusion, pour 1 cup boiling water over 1–2 teaspoons (5–10 mL) dried herb; infuse 10–15 minutes. Drink 3 times per day.

When using the tincture, take 1–4 mL 3 times per day.

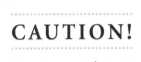

CAUTION!

Do not use motherwort during pregnancy.

NIGHT-BLOOMING CEREUS (*Selenicereus grandiflorus*, Britt. & Rose, Cactaceae)

Part Used: Flowers, young stems.
Actions: Cardiotonic.
Indications: This unique herb was once used extensively for a wide range of cardiologic problems. However, it is now in very short supply because of environmental degradation of its habitat. Unfortunately, some of the material sold as "cactus" is another genus of cactus altogether. I wonder about the tinctures that now appear on the market. This is a case where taxonomic exactitude is essential.

The main reason why night-blooming cereus is no longer used in orthodox medicine (although it is discussed in pharmacology books) largely concerns convenience and economics. The plant does not contain a cardiac glycoside. It works in a unique way that has not received enough research. It seems to stimulate the action of the heart, increasing the strength of contractions while slowing the heart rate. Night-blooming cereus has been used for conditions such as angina pectoris and congestive heart failure. Perhaps its most important contribution is as a heart tonic during the crucial recuperative period after a heart attack.

Preparation and Dosage: Use only if you are under professional supervision.

OATS (*Avena sativa*, L. Poaceae)

Part Used: Seeds and whole plant.

Actions: Nervine tonic, antidepressant, nutritive, demulcent, vulnerary.

Indications: Oats is one of the best herbs for "feeding" the nervous system, especially under conditions of stress. It is considered to be a specific in cases of nervous debility and exhaustion associated with depression. Oats may be used with most of the other nervines, both relaxant and stimulatory, to strengthen the whole of the nervous system. It is also used in cases of general debility. The high levels of silicic acid in the straw explain the usefulness of oats as a remedy for skin conditions, especially when applied externally.

Preparation and Dosage: To make an infusion, pour 1 cup boiling water over 1–3 teaspoons (5–15 mL) dried straw; infuse 10–15 minutes. Drink 3 times per day.

When using a tincture, take ¾–1 teaspoon (3–5 mL) 3 times per day.

When using oats in the bath for neuralgia and irritated skin conditions, boil 1 pound shredded straw in 2 quarts water for 30 minutes. Strain the liquid and add it to the bath. You can also put the cooked, rolled oats in a muslin bag and put the bag in the bath water.

PARSLEY (*Petroselinum crispum,* [Mill] Nyman ex. A. W. Hill, Apiaceae)

Part Used: Leaves, seeds.

Actions: Diuretic, expectorant, emmenagogue, carminative, antispasmodic, hypotensive.

Indications: The fresh herb, so widely used in cooking, is a rich source of vitamin C. Medicinally, parsley has three main areas of use. First, it is an effective diuretic, helping the body get rid of excess water. (Keep in mind, however, that the underlying cause of the problem must be treated — don't just treat the symptoms.) Second, it's an emmenagogue, stimulating the menstrual process. Third, it's a carminative, easing flatulence and the colic pains that may accompany it.

Preparation and Dosage: To make an infusion, pour 1 cup boiling water over 1–2 teaspoons (5–10 mL) leaves or root; infuse 5–10 minutes in a closed container. Drink 3 times per day.

When using a tincture, take 1–2 mL 3 times per day.

> # CAUTION!
>
> Do not use parsley if you are pregnant, as it may cause excessive stimulation of the uterus. Do not use parsley if you have kidney disease.

PASSIONFLOWER (*Passiflora incarnata,* Passifloraceae)

Part Used: Leaves and whole plant.

Actions: Nervine, hypnotic, antispasmodic, anodyne, hypotensive.

Indications: Passionflower depresses central nervous system activity and is hypotensive. It is used for its sedative and soothing properties — to lower blood pressure, prevent tachycardia, and relieve insomnia. The alkaloids and flavonoids have been reported to have sedative effects in animals. Many of the flavonoids, such as apigenin, are well-known for pharmacologic activity, particularly antispasmodic and anti-inflammatory activities.

Passionflower is the herb of choice for treating intransigent insomnia. It aids the transition into restful sleep without any "narcotic" hangover. It may be used whenever an antispasmodic is required: for example, in Parkinson's disease, seizures, and hysteria. It can be very effective for nerve pain, such as neuralgia, and for shingles, a viral infection of nerves. It may also be used for asthma, a condition with much spasmodic activity, and especially for asthma with associated tension.

Preparation and Dosage: To make an infusion, pour 1 cup boiling water over 1 teaspoon (5 mL) dried herb; infuse 15 minutes. Drink a cup in the evening for sleeplessness and a cup twice per day to ease other conditions.

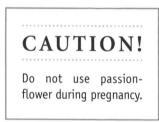

CAUTION!

Do not use passionflower during pregnancy.

When using a tincture, take 1–4 mL in the evening for sleeplessness and 1–4 mL twice per day to ease other conditions.

PRICKLY ASH (*Zanthoxylum americanum*, Mill. Rutaceae)

Part Used: Bark, berries.

Actions: Stimulant (circulatory), tonic, alterative, carminative, diaphoretic, antirheumatic, hepatic.

Indications: Use of prickly ash is similar to that of cayenne, although prickly ash acts more slowly. Prickly ash is indicated for many chronic problems, such as rheumatism and skin diseases. Any sign of poor circulation — for example, chilblains, leg cramps, varicose veins, and varicose ulcers — calls for use of this herb. Externally, prickly ash may be used as a stimulating liniment for rheumatism and fibrositis. Because of its stimulating effect on the lymphatic system, circulation, and mucous membranes, it has a role in the holistic treatment of many specific conditions.

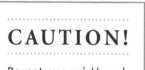

CAUTION!

Do not use prickly ash during pregnancy.

Preparation and Dosage: To make an infusion, pour 1 cup boiling water over 1–2 teaspoons (5–10 mL) dried herb; infuse 10–15 minutes. Drink 3 times per day.

When using a tincture, take 1–2 mL 3 times per day.

ROSEMARY (*Rosmarinus officinalis*, L. Lamiaceae)

Part Used: Leaves, twigs.

Actions: Carminative, antispasmodic, antidepressive, rubefacient, antimicrobial, emmenagogue.

Indications: Rosemary is a circulatory and nervine stimulant. It also has a toning and calming effect on digestion when psychological tension is present. It may be used for flatulent dyspepsia, headache, or depression associated with debility. Externally, it may be used to ease muscular pain, sciatica, and neuralgia. It acts as a stimulant to both the hair follicles and circulation in the scalp, which may be helpful for premature baldness.

Preparation and Dosage: To make an infusion, pour 1 cup boiling water over 1–2 teaspoons (5–10 mL) dried herb; infuse in a covered container 10–15 minutes. Drink 3 times per day.

When using a tincture, take 1–2 mL 3 times per day.

SCOTS BROOM (*Cytisus scoparius*, [L.] Link., Fabaceae)

Part Used: Flowering tops.

Actions: Cardioactive, diuretic, hypertensive, peripheral vasoconstrictor, astringent.

Indications: Broom is a valuable remedy for a weak heart and low blood pressure. Because it is also a diuretic and produces peripheral constriction of the blood vessels while increasing the efficiency of each stroke of the heart, it can be used when water is retained as a result of heart weakness. Broom is also used for overprofuse menstruation.

> **CAUTION!**
>
> Do not use Scots broom during pregnancy or if you have hypertension.

Preparation and Dosage: To make an infusion, pour 1 cup boiling water over 1 teaspoon (5 mL) dried herb; infuse 10–15 minutes. Drink 3 times per day.

When using a tincture, take 1–2 mL 3 times per day.

SIBERIAN GINSENG (*Eleutherococcus senticosus,* Araliaceae)

Part Used: Root.

Actions: Adaptogen.

Indications: Siberian ginseng can be recommended as a general tonic for a wide range of clinical indications. It is especially useful for conditions affected by the stress response, including angina, hypertension, hypotension, chronic bronchitis, and cancer. It is also helpful for treating the effects of prolonged stress or over-work, such as exhaustion, irritability, insomnia, and mild depression. It can be used to assist in recovery from acute or chronic diseases, trauma, surgery, and other stressful episodes or to counter the debilitating effects of chronic disease and treatments such as chemotherapy and radiation. It can be taken on a long-term basis to minimize the incidence of acute infections and to improve well-being.

Preparation and Dosage: According to clinical studies, the standard dosage of the tincture is 50–100 drops 3 times per day (or 100–200 mg of a solid extract concentrated at a ratio of 20:1). The recommended regimen involves using the tincture for 6 weeks and then taking a 2-week break.

CAUTION!

Consult a medical professional before using Siberian ginseng during pregnancy or administering it to children.

SKULLCAP (*Scutellaria laterifolia,* L. Lamiaceae)

Part Used: Aerial parts.

Actions: Nervine tonic, antispasmodic, hypotensive.

Indications: Skullcap may be the most useful nervine available. It relaxes states of nervous tension while renewing and revivifying the central nervous system. It has a specific use in the treatment of seizure and hysterical states as well as epilepsy. Skullcap may be used to treat all exhausted or depressed conditions. It can be used with complete safety for easing premenstrual tension.

Preparation and Dosage: To make an infusion, pour 1 cup boiling water over 1–2 teaspoons (5–10 mL) dried herb; infuse 10–15 minutes. Drink 3 times per day or as needed.

When using the tincture, take 2–4 mL 3 times per day.

St.-John's-Wort (*Hypericum perforatum,* Guttiferae)

Parts Used: Aerial parts.

Actions: Anti-inflammatory, astringent, vulnerary, nervine, antimicrobial.

Indications: Taken internally, St.-John's-wort has a sedative and pain-reducing effect. It's helpful for treating neuralgia, anxiety, tension, and similar problems and is especially useful for menopausal changes triggering irritability and anxiety. It is increasingly recommended for treating depression and can also be used to ease fibrositis, sciatica, and rheumatic pain. Externally, it is a valuable healing and anti-inflammatory remedy. As a lotion, it speeds healing of wounds and bruises, varicose veins, and mild burns. The oil is especially useful for the healing of sunburn.

Preparation and Dosage: To make an infusion, pour 1 cup boiling water over 1–2 teaspoons (5–10 mL) dried herb; infuse 10–15 minutes. Drink 3 times per day.

When using a tincture, take 2–4 mL 3 times per day.

CAUTION!

Do not use St.-John's-wort if you are also using an antidepressant medication. May cause photosensitivity, especially in fair-skinned people.

VALERIAN (*Valeriana officinalis,* L. Valarianaceae)

Part Used: Rhizome.
Actions: Nervine, hypnotic, antispasmodic, carminative, hypotensive, emmenagogue.
Indications: Valerian has a wide range of specific uses but is primarily applied for anxiety; nervous sleeplessness; and physical signs of tension, such as muscle cramps or indigestion. For some people, it acts as a mild pain reliever. It's also an effective herbal sleep remedy, with the advantage that it is not powerful enough to interfere with necessary REM sleep. Valerian is an effective muscle relaxant and can be used for all kinds of cramps, including uterine cramps and intestinal colic. Its sedative and antispasmodic action can be partially ascribed to the valepotriates and, to a lesser extent, the sesquiterpene constituents of the volatile oils. Species of valerian are used worldwide as relaxing remedies for hypertension and stress-related heart problems.
Dosage and Preparation: The tincture is the most widely used preparation. The recommended dosage is 2.5–5 mL (½–1 teaspoon), although some situations may require up to 10 ml. Take as needed.

To make an infusion, pour 8 ounces cold water over 2 teaspoons (10 mL) dried root; let stand 8–10 hours. This yields one dose that can be taken in the morning (when allowed to stand overnight) and then again in the evening (when allowed to stand during the day).

WILD CARROT (*Daucus carrota,* L. Apiaceae)

Parts Used: Dried aerial parts and seeds.
Actions: Diuretic, antilithic, carminative, antispasmodic.
Indications: The volatile oil present in wild carrot is an active urinary antiseptic; this helps explain its use for conditions like cystitis and prostatitis. It has long been considered a specific in the treatment of kidney stones. For treating gout and rheumatism, wild

carrot is combined with other remedies to provide a cleansing diuretic action. The seeds can be used as a settling carminative agent to relieve flatulence and colic.

Preparation and Dosage: To make an infusion, pour 1 cup boiling water over 1 teaspoon (5 mL) dried herb; infuse 10–15 minutes. Drink 3 times per day. To prepare an infusion of the seeds, use ⅓ to 1 teaspoon seeds to 1 cup water.

When using a tincture, take 1–2 mL 3 times per day.

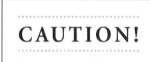

CAUTION!

Do not use wild carrot seeds during pregnancy.

WITCH HAZEL (*Hamamelis virginiana*, L. Hamamelidaceae)

Part Used: Leaves and twigs
Actions: Astringent, anti-inflammatory.
Indications: This herb can be found in most households in the form of distilled witch hazel. It is the most applicable and easy-to-use astringent. As with all astringents, it may be used wherever bleeding has occurred, internally or externally. It is especially useful for easing hemorrhoids. Witch hazel has a deserved reputation for treating bruises and inflamed swellings as well as varicose veins. It controls diarrhea and helps ease dysentery.
Preparation and Dosage: To make an infusion, pour 1 cup boiling water over 1 teaspoon (5 mL) dried leaves; infuse 10–15 minutes. Drink 3 times per day.

When using a tincture, take 1–2 mL 3 times per day.

WOOD BETONY (*Stachys officinalis*, L. Lamiaceae)

Parts Used: Dried aerial parts.
Actions: Nervine, bitter.
Indications: Wood betony gently tones and strengthens the nervous system but also relaxes. It can help relieve nervous debility associated with anxiety and tension. It is also good for headaches

and neuralgia of a nervous origin as well as those caused by hypertension.

Combinations: For the treatment of nervous headache, wood betony combines well with skullcap. It can be combined with the appropriate hypotensives for treating hypertensive headaches.

Preparation and Dosage: To make an infusion, pour 1 cup boiling water over 1–2 teaspoons (5–10 mL) dried herb; infuse 10–15 minutes. Drink 3 times per day.

When using a tincture, take 2–6 mL 3 times per day.

YARROW (*Achillea millefolium*, L. Asteraceae)

Parts Used: Aerial parts.

Actions: Diaphoretic, hypotensive, astringent, anti-inflammatory, diuretic, antimicrobial, bitter, hepatic.

Indications: Yarrow is one of the best diaphoretic herbs and is a standard remedy for fever. It reduces blood pressure through dilatation of the peripheral vessels. It stimulates digestion and tones the blood vessels. As a urinary antiseptic, yarrow is indicated for infections such as cystitis. Used externally, it helps heal wounds. It is considered to be a specific in thrombotic conditions associated with hypertension.

Preparation and Dosage: To make an infusion, pour 1 cup boiling water over 1–2 teaspoons (5–10 mL) dried herb; infuse 10–15 minutes. Drink hot 3 times per day. When you are feverish, drink hourly.

When using a tincture, take 2–4 mL 3 times per day.

CAUTION!

Do not use yarrow during pregnancy. May produce photosensitivity and allergic reactions in sensitive people.

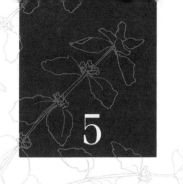

MAKING HERBAL
MEDICINE

There is no mystery to making healing formulations from plants, and you don't need to be particularly clever. The pharmaceutical elite would have us think that to be of any use, a medicine must be made by a Ph.D. wearing a white lab coat and must then be packaged with half an acre of rain forest material. Not so! If you can make a cup of tea and cook a meal that your friends would be willing to eat, you are qualified to make herbal medicine.

Various methods of using plants have been developed over the centuries. No doubt, our ancestors first used herbs by eating the fresh plants. Since then, over the thousands of years that herbs have been used, other methods of preparing them have been developed. With our modern knowledge of pharmacology, we can make conscious choices about the process we use to release the biochemical constituents that are all-important to healing — without insulting the integrity of the plant by isolating fractions of the whole.

The most effective way to use herbs is to take them internally, since healing takes place from within. The ways of preparing internal remedies are numerous, but it is essential to take care with the process to ensure that you end up with what you want.

TEAS

Water-based herbal extracts are called *infusions* and *decoctions*. Following is the basic rule for choosing which method to use with which herb.

In general, an infusion is the appropriate preparation method for nonwoody materials, such as leaves, flowers, and some stems. A decoction is preferable if the herb contains hard or woody material, such as roots, barks, or nuts. The denser the plant or its individual cell walls, the more energy is needed to extract the cell contents into the tea. Thus, decoction is the more effective method for extracting the contents of dense plant matter.

As with anything in the real world, there are exceptions to this guideline. For instance, roots that are rich in volatile oil, such as valerian root, are better infused than decocted. For, while the woodiness of the root suggests that decocting is appropriate, when the roots are simmered, the therapeutically important volatile oil boils off.

How to Make an Infusion

If you know how to make tea, you know how to make an infusion. An infusion is the simplest way to use both fresh and dried herbs. However, since fresh and dried herbs differ in water content, when one part dried herb is prescribed, it should be replaced with three parts fresh herb. For instance, if a recipe calls for 1 teaspoon dried herb, 3 teaspoons fresh herb can be substituted.

Step 1. Warm a china or glass teapot by pouring hot water into the pot, letting it sit a few minutes, and then emptying. Place dried herb in the pot, about 1 teaspoon for each cup of tea.

Step 2. Pour 1 cup boiling water for each teaspoon of herb into the teapot; put the lid on. Allow to steep 10–15 minutes.

Sweeten to taste. It's usually best to drink medicinal herb infusions hot, but they can also be drunk cold.

THE BEST HERBS FOR INFUSION

Many herbal infusions make exquisite additions to one's lifestyle and can open up a whole world of subtle delights and pleasures. Infusions are not only medicines or "alternatives" to coffee but are also excellent beverages in their own right. Everyone has his or her favorite herbs, and here are some of my favorite-tasting teas. These herbs may be used singly or in combination, and your selection can be based on both taste and medicinal properties.

Flowers: Chamomile, elder flower, hibiscus, linden blossom, red clover

Leaves: Peppermint, spearmint, lemon balm, rosemary, lemon verbena

Berries: Hawthorn, rose hips

Seeds: Aniseed, caraway, celery, dill, fennel

Roots: Licorice

Tea bags. You can make your own tea bags by filling little muslin bags with the dried herb. Take care to remember how many teaspoons have been put into each bag so you know how much water to add. Use these tea bags just as you would use ordinary teabags.

Large quantities. Larger quantities of infusion can be made in the proportion of 1 ounce herb to 1 pint water. Store in the refrigerator, since the shelf life of an infusion is not very long; any microorganism that enters the infusion will multiply and thrive in it. At the first sign of fermentation or spoilage, discard the infusion. Whenever possible, infusions should be prepared fresh.

Preparing the herb. Infusions are best for nonwoody parts of the plant, where the active ingredients are easily accessible. If an infusion is to be made of bark, root, seeds, or resin, it is best to powder these parts first to break down some of the cell walls; this makes the cells more accessible to water. Seeds, such as fennel and aniseed, should be slightly bruised before infusing to release the volatile oils from the cells. Any aromatic herb should be infused in a well-sealed pot to ensure that a minimum of the volatile oil is lost through evaporation.

Cold infusion. If the herbs are sensitive to heat, either because they contain highly volatile oils or because their constituents break down at high temperatures, make a cold infusion. The proportion of herb to water is the same, but the infusion should be left for 6 to 12 hours in a well-sealed pot of cool water. When it is ready, strain and drink.

How to Make a Decoction

If the herbs you've selected are hard and woody, a decoction will ensure that the soluble contents of the herbs actually reach the water. Roots, rhizomes, wood, bark, nuts, and some seeds are hard, with very strong cell walls. To ensure that the constituents of the materials are transferred to the water, more heat than the amount used for infusions is needed.

Step 1. In a heatproof glass, ceramic, earthenware, or enameled metal saucepan, place 1 teaspoon dried herb for each cup water. If larger quantities are desired, use 1 ounce dried herb for each pint water.

Step 2. Add 1 cup water for each teaspoon dried herb. Bring to a boil, reduce heat, and simmer 10–15 minutes or the amount of time specified for the particular herb or mixture. If the herb contains volatile oils, put a lid on the pot.

Step 3. Strain the tea while still hot and drink.

If you're preparing a mixture that contains both soft and woody herbs, prepare a separate infusion with the soft herbs and then combine with the decoction before drinking. For a woody herb that is rich in volatile herbs, it is best to powder the herb finely and make an infusion rather than making a decoction (since the oils would boil away).

TINCTURES

Extracts of herbs in alcohol are called *tinctures*. Alcohol is a better solvent than water for most plant constituents, and the alcohol (mixed with water) dissolves nearly all the plant's ingredients and acts as a preservative. Occasionally glycerin is used as a base for a tincture, but most are made with alcohol.

How to Make a Tincture

The method outlined here is a basic approach. Professionally prepared tinctures use specific water/alcohol proportions for each herb, but for the herbs described in this book, the following general directions are fine. If you are using fresh rather than dried herbs, use twice the amount.

Step 1. In a container that can be tightly closed, place 4 ounces finely chopped or ground dried herb. (For fresh herbs, use twice as much herb.) Pour 1 pint 60-proof vodka over the herbs and close tightly with a lid.

Step 2. Place the container in a warm, dark place for 2 weeks, shaking it once a day.

Step 3. Pour off the bulk of the liquid, then strain the remaining liquid through a muslin cloth suspended in a bowl. Wring out all the liquid from the herbs. The spent herbs make excellent compost!

Step 4. Pour the tincture into a dark bottle. Label bottle and keep tightly closed with a lid or stopper.

Because tinctures are much stronger, volume for volume, than infusions or decoctions, the dosage is usually much smaller.

Uses: Tinctures may be used in a variety of ways. They can be taken straight or mixed with water. If a tincture is added to hot water, the alcohol in the tincture will largely evaporate, leaving most of the extract in the water. A few drops of tincture can also be added to a bath or footbath, used in a compress, or mixed with oil and fat to make an ointment. Suppositories and lozenges can also be made from tinctures.

Other Bases for Tinctures

Another way to make an alcohol tincture is to infuse herbs in wine. Even though these wine-based preparations do not have the shelf life of tinctures and are less concentrated, they can be both pleasant to take and effective.

The advantages of glycerin-based tinctures is that they are milder on the digestive tract and do not involve the problems associated with alcohol. However, the disadvantage is that glycerin does not dissolve resinous or oily plant material well. As a solvent, glycerin is generally better than water but not as good as alcohol.

DRY HERB PREPARATIONS

Taking herbs in dry form has many advantages. The primary one is that the taste of the herb can be avoided while the whole herb (including the woody material) is consumed. Unfortunately, taking herbs in dry form also has several drawbacks.

- Dry herbs are unprocessed, so the constituents are not always readily available for easy absorption. During infusion, heat and water help break down the walls of the plant cells and dissolve the constituents; however, the digestive process of the stomach and small intestines is not guaranteed to break down plant cell walls.
- When the constituents are already dissolved in liquid form, they are available much faster and begin their action sooner.
- A subtler drawback is that you do not taste the herb. Some herbs, such as the bitters, work best when tasted because their effects result from a neurological reflex. When bitters are put into a capsule or pill, their action may be lost or diminished.

Two ways to use herbs in dry form are in capsules and pills. Be sure that the herbs are powdered as finely as possible. Grinding guarantees that the cell walls are largely broken down and helps you digest and absorb the herb.

Capsules

A convenient way to take powdered herbs is in gelatin capsules. The capsule size needed depends on the amount of herbs prescribed per dose, the density of the plant, and the volume of the material. A size "00" capsule, for instance, holds about ⅙ ounce of finely powdered herb.

Filling a capsule is easy:

Step 1. Place the powdered herbs on a flat dish and separate the halves of the capsule.

Step 2. Move the halves of the capsule through the powder, scooping the herb into the two halves.

Step 3. Push the halves of the capsule together.

Pills

Pills can be made in many ways, ranging from the very simple to the complex. The simplest way is to sprinkle the herb powder onto a piece of fresh bread and then roll it into a small ball. This works most effectively with herbs that are unpleasant to take, such as cayenne.

INDEX

Entries in **bold** indicate recipes; page references in *italics* indicate illustrations.

Adaptogens, 35, 104
  defined, 24
Alcohol consumption
  beneficial effects, 11
  hypertension, 46, 53
  vasodilating effects, 11
Alteratives, 35, 85, 102
  defined, 24
Angelica
  digestive system effects, 29
  respiratory system effects, 29
Angina pectoris, 66
  hawthorn for treatment, 67
  symptoms, 66–68
  therapeutic approaches, 68
Angina Tincture, 67
Antihypertensives, side effects, 55
Anti-inflammatories, 32, 33, 35, 78,
    80, 81, 82, 84, 87, 89, 91, 94, 105,
    107, 108
  defined, 24
Antimicrobials, 32, 33, 35, 82
  defined, 24
Antispasmodics, 35, 49, 71, 80, 82, 85,
    87, 88, 91, 93, 94, 95, 98, 101, 103,
    104, 106
  atherosclerosis, 59
  defined, 24
  intermittent claudication, 69–70
Arnica (*Arnica montana*,
    L. Asteraceae), *78–79*
  toxicity, 79
Arteries, hardening of. *See*
    Atherosclerosis
Arteriosclerosis, 15, 47, 55.
See also Atherosclerosis
Atherosclerosis, 55–61
  blood pressure, 58

  cholesterol, 57–58
  diet, 58
  exercise, 58
  herbal treatment, 59
  lifestyle, 61
  obesity, 58
  progression, 57
  risk factors, 57
  sodium intake, 60
  vitamin supplements, 60, 61
Atherosclerosis Tincture, 59

"**B**ad cholesterol." *See* Low-density
    lipoprotein
Balm, relaxing effect of, 30
Beta blockers, 36, 41
Bilberry, cardiotonic effects of, 28
Birth control pills, 9–10
  blood pressure, 10
  See also Oral contraceptives
Blood clots, 15, 56
  garlic to reduce, 18
Blood pressure
  heart disease, 11–12
  measuring, 44
  See also Hypertension
Bugleweed (*Lycopus europaeus,*
    L. Lamiaceae), *79*
  circulatory system effects, 29

Caffeine, 31
  hypertension, 53
Calcium-channel blockers, 41–42
Calcium supplements, 53
Capsules, making, 115
Caraway, to lower cholesterol, 17
Cardiac glycosides, 1–3, 27, 36–38
  congestive heart failure, 64

Cardiac remedies, 2–3, 26–30
  defined, 25, 26
Cardioactives, 2, 34, 36–39, 94, 104
  description, 27
Cardiotonics, 2–4, 35–37, 48, 80, 98,
    99, 103
  atherosclerosis, 59
  circulatory system, 29
  congestive heart failure, 64
  defined, 26
  description, 27
  digestive system, 29
  intermittent claudication, 69–70
  musculoskeletal system, 29
  nervous system, 30
  reproductive system, 29
  respiratory system, 29
  See also Cardiac remedies
Cathinone, 40
Cayenne (*Capsicum frutescens*,
    L. Solanaceae), *79–80*
  circulatory stimulant action, 29
  lowering cholesterol, 17
Chamomile. *See* German chamomile
Cholesterol, 14–19
  arteriosclerosis, 15
  blood levels, 15–16
  lowering, 16–20
  See also High-density lipoprotein;
    Low-density lipoprotein
Circulation problems, 71–72
  causes, 71
  herbal treatment, 71–72
  therapeutic approaches, 72
Circulatory stimulants, 49, 71, 95, 102
  atherosclerosis, 59
Circulatory system, *44*
Claudication. *See* Intermittent claudi-
    cation
Cleavers (*Galium aparine*,
    L. Rubiaceae), *80*
Clots. *See* Blood clots
Coenzyme Q_{10}, 20–22
  atherosclerosis, 61
  congestive heart failure, 65

  deficiency and heart failure, 21
  hypertension, 54
  sources, 21
Coleus (*Coleus forskohlii,* Lamiaceae),
    39, *80–81*
Congestive heart failure, 62–66
  coenzyme Q_{10} deficiency, 21
  herbal treatment, 64
  risk factors, 62–63
  symptoms, 63
Congestive Heart Failure Formula, 65
Corn (*Zea mays,* L. Poaceae), *81*
Cornsilk, 31
Coronary artery disease, 56
Couchgrass (*Elytrigia repens* ssp.
    repens, [L.] Beauvois, Poaceae), 31,
    82
Cramp bark (*Viburnum opulus,*
    L. Caprifoliaceae), 49, *82–83*
  hypotensive action, 48

Dandelion (*Taraxacum officinale,*
    Asteraceae), 31, *83*
  circulatory system, effects on, 32
Decoctions, making, 112
Diabetes
  atherosclerosis, 58
  heart disease, 12–13
Diaphoretics, 34, 35
  defined, 25
Diet, 10, 18–22
  congestive heart failure, 65
  guidelines, 20–22
  hypertension, 54
  varicose veins, 76–77
  vegetarian, 54
Digitalis, diuretic action of, 38
Digoxin, 27
Diuretics, 30–33, 35, 49, 79, 80, 81, 82,
    83, 85, 89, 93, 94, 101, 103, 106, 108
  congestive heart failure, 64
  defined, 25, 30
  herbs containing, 31
  intermittent claudication, 69–70
  secondary effects, 32–34

Edema, defined, 30
Emblica officinalis
    lowering cholesterol, 17
Ephedrine, in plants, 39
Epicatechin, 28
Exercise, 61
    blood circulation, 72
    congestive heart failure, 65
    trigger for angina, 67

Fat
    congestive heart failure, 65
    reducing, 20
Fenugreek, to lower cholesterol, 17
Feverfew (*Chrysanthemum parthenium*, [L.] Bernh. Asteraceae), 84–85
    cautions, 84
Figwort (*Scrophularia nodosa*, Juss. Scrophulariaceae), 85
    circulatory system effects, 29
Flavonoids, 4, 28, 41
    heart disease, 38
Flaxseed oil, and atherosclerosis, 61
Folic acid, sources of, 22
Formula for Hypertension-Related Palpitations, 51
Forskolin, 39
Foxglove, 1–2, 27, 31
    circulatory system effects, 29
    toxicity, 28, 37

Garlic (*Allium sativum*, L. Liliaceae), 85–86
    angina, 68
    atherosclerosis, 61
    blood clots, 18
    cholesterol, 17, 40
    circulatory system effects, 29
    digestive system effects, 29
    hypertension, 48, 54
    respiratory system effects, 29
Gentian (*Gentiana lutea*, L. Gentianaceae), 86–87

German chamomile (*Matricaria recutita*, L. Asteraceae), 87–88
Ginger (*Zingiber officinale*, Roscoe Zingiberaceae), 88–89
    cautions, 88
    circulatory stimulant action, 29
Gingko (*Ginkgo biloba*, L. Ginkgoaceae), 49, 89
    circulatory system effects, 29
    treatment uses, 7
"Good cholesterol." *See* High-density lipoprotein
Guarana, 31
Gugulipid (*Commiphora mukul*), 17

Hawthorn (*Crataegus laevigata* and *C. monogyna*, L. Rosaceae), 89–90
    circulatory system effects, 29
Hawthorn Berry Conserve, 90
Hawthorn, 3, 49
    active constituents, 4–5
    angina treatment, 67
    cardiotonic effects, 28
    clinical studies, 5
    hypotensive action, 48
    intermittent claudication, 69
Heart, enlarged, 47
Heart attacks, 47
Heart failure
    classification levels, 6
See also Congestive heart failure
Heart stimulant, 85
Hepatics, 34, 35, 83, 86, 98, 102, 108
    defined, 26
Herbs, dry preparations, 114–115
Heredity, and cardiovascular disease, 10
High blood pressure. *See* Hypertension
High-density lipoprotein (HDL), 15–17
    increasing, 19
Homocysteine levels in blood, 21

Horsechestnut (*Aesculus hippocas-
tanum*, L. Hippocastanaceae), 91
  caution, 91
  circulatory system effects, 29
Horseradish, circulatory stimulant
  action of, 29
Hypertension, 43–55
  African Americans, 44
  atherosclerosis, 58
  causes, 46
  complications, 47
  congestive heart failure, 65
  dietary supplements, 54
  dietary therapies, 54
  lifestyle therapies, 54–55
  risk factors, 46
  symptoms, 46–47
  weight, 54
  See also Hypotensives
Hypertension Formula, 50
**Hypertension with Headache
  Formula, 51**
Hypertensives, 95, 103
Hypotensives, 34, 41–42, 48–51, 80,
  82, 93, 94, 98, 101, 104, 106
  atherosclerosis, 59
  congestive heart failure, 64
  defined, 26
  intermittent claudication, 69–70
  secondary actions, 35

Infusions, making, 110–112
**Intermittent Claudication Formula,
  70**
Intermittent claudication, 69–70
  herbal treatment, 69–70
  symptoms, 69

Kava kava (*Piper methysticum*,
  G. Forst. Piperaceae), 91–92
  caution, 92
Khat, 40
Kidney damage, 47
Kola (*Cola acuminata*, [Beauv.] Schott
  & Endl., Sterculiaceae), 31, 93

Lavender (*Lavandula angustifolia*,
  Miller, Lamiaceae), *93*
L-carnitine, and congestive heart
  failure, 65
Ligustrum lucidum, lowering cholesterol, 17
Lily of the valley (*Convallaria majalis*,
  Liliaceae), 1–2, 28, *94*
  circulatory system effects, 29, 32
Linden (*Tilia spp.*, Tiliaceae), 49, *94*
  circulatory system effects, 29
  digestive system effects, 29
  relaxing effect, 30
Lobelia (*Lobelia inflata*,
  L. Campanulaceae), *95*
  caution, 95
Low-density lipoprotein (LDL),
  15–16, 18
  atherosclerosis risk, 57

Ma huang (*Ephedra sinica*, Staph.
  Ephedraceae), 39, 95–96
  caution, 97
  contraindications, 7
  side effects, 96–97
Magnesium
  atherosclerosis, 61
  blood circulation, 72
  congestive heart failure, 65
  hypertension, 54
  supplements, 53
  varicose veins, 77
Milk thistle (*Silybum marianum*,
  [L.] Gaertn. Asteraceae), *98*
Monounsaturated fats, increasing,
  18–19
Motherwort (*Leonurus cardiaca*,
  L. Lamiaceae), 49, *98–99*
  caution, 99
  circulatory system effects, 29
  digestive system effects, 29
  relaxing effect, 30
Mustard, circulatory stimulant action
  of, 29

Nervines, 34, 35, 49, 79, 82, 87, 91, 95, 98, 100, 101, 104, 105, 106, 107
  atherosclerosis, 59
  congestive heart failure, 64
  defined, 26
  intermittent claudication, 70
Niacin, and atherosclerosis, 61
Night-blooming cereus (*Selenicereus grandiflorus,* Britt. & Rose, Cactaceae), 99–100
  cardiotonic effects, 28
Nitrogen-containing compounds, 40

Oats (*Avena sativa,* L. Poaceae), *100*
Obesity
  atherosclerosis, 58
  heart disease, 12
  hypertension, 53
  varicose veins, 73
Oligomeric proanthocyanidin (OPC) 4, 5
Onions
  angina, 68
  blood pressure, 18
  cholesterol, 17
Oral contraceptives, 9–10
  heart disease risk, 9
  hypertension, 54
  smoking, 9
  See also Birth control pills

Parsley (*Petroselinum crispum,* [Mill] Nyman ex. A. W. Hill, Apiaceae), *101*
  caution, 100
Passionflower (*Passiflora incarnata,* Passifloraceae), *101*–102
  caution, 102
Personality typing, 13
Phenylalkylamines, 39–40
Phytosterols, 16
  cholesterol, 40
  heart disease, 38
Pills, making, 115

Plaques, 15
  defined, 56
  garlic to reduce, 18
Polygonatum sibiricum, *39*
Potassium, 52
Prickly ash (*Zanthoxylum americanum,* Mill. Rutaceae), *102*–103
  cardiotonic effects, 28
  caution, 102
  circulatory stimulant action, 29
Prostaglandin, for lowering blood pressure, 18
Psyllium seeds, as a fiber source, 20

Riboflavin (Vitamin B_2), 21
Risk factors for heart disease, 8–22
Rosemary (*Rosmarinus officinalis,* L. Lamiaceae), *103*
  digestive system effects, 29
  relaxing effect, 30

Salt. *See* Sodium
Saturated fats
  hypertension, 53
  reducing, 19
Scots broom (*Cytisus scoparius,* [L.] Link., Fabaceae), 31, 103–104
  cardiotonic effects, 28
  caution, 103
  circulatory system effects, 29, 32
  contraindications, 7
Siberian ginseng (*Eleutherococcus senticosus,* Araliaceae), *104*
  caution, 104
Skullcap (*Scutellaria laterifolia,* L. Lamiaceae), 49, *104*–105
Smoking
  angina, 67
  atherosclerosis, 58
  death rate, 10
  heart disease, 9, 10
  hypertension, 46
Sodium
  atherosclerosis, 60

blood pressure, 52
congestive heart failure, 65
Squill, circulatory system effects, 29
St.-John's-wort (*Hypericum perfora-
tum,* Guttiferae), 105
caution, 105
Stress, 13–14
**Stress-Related Hypertension
Formula, 50**
Stroke, 47
Sugar, and hypertension, 53
Sulfur compounds, and lower heart
disease, 38
Supplements
congestive heart failure, 65
guidelines, 19–22
Sympathomimetics, 36, 39
Synephrine, 40

Tea, 31, 110
Tinctures, making 113–114
Tonics, 34, 35, 80, 81, 83, 102
defined, 26
Triglycerides, 15

Ubiquinone. *See* Coenzyme Q_{10}
Uva-ursi, 31

Valerian (*Valeriana officinalis,*
L. Valerianaceae), 49, *106*
Varicose Vein Formula, 75
Varicose Vein Lotion, 75
Varicose veins, 73
contributing factors, 73–74
defined, 73
herbal treatment, 74
supplements, 76–77
therapeutic approaches, 74, 76–77
Vascular tonics, 49, 71
atherosclerosis, 59
Vasoconstrictors, 79, 103
Vasodilators, 49, 71, 80, 84, 89, 95
atherosclerosis, 59

congestive heart failure, 64
intermittent claudication, 69–70
Very-low-density lipoprotein (VLDL),
15
Vitamin A, and varicose veins, 77
Vitamin B complex, and varicose
veins, 77
Vitamin B_{12}, sources, 22
Vitamin B_2, 21
Vitamin B_3, 72
Vitamin B_6, sources, 22
Vitamin C, 21
atherosclerosis, 61
blood circulation, 72
hypertension, 54
varicose veins, 77
Vitamin E, 21
atherosclerosis, 61
blood circulation, 72
hypertension, 54
varicose veins, 77
Vulneraries, 35, 78, 87, 100, 105
defined, 26

Weight
angina, 68
atherosclerosis, 60
hypertension, 54
Wild carrot (*Daucus carrota,*
L. Apiaceae), *106–107*
caution, 107
Witch hazel (*Hamamelis virginiana,*
L. Hamamelidaceae), *107*
Wood betony (*Stachys officinalis,*
L. Lamiaceae), *107–108*

Yarrow (*Achillea millefolium,*
L. Asteraceae), 49, *108*
caution, 108
circulatory system effects, 29, 32

Zinc, and varicose veins, 77

OTHER STOREY TITLES YOU WILL ENJOY

Easy Breathing, by David Hoffmann. 128 pages. Paperback. ISBN 1-58017-252-0.

Healthy Digestion, by David Hoffmann. 128 pages. Paperback. ISBN 1-58017-250-4.

Healthy Bones and Joints, by David Hoffmann. 128 pages. Paperback. ISBN 1-58017-253-9.

Herbs for Hepatitis C and the Liver, by Stephen Harrod Buhner. 128 pages. Paperback. ISBN 1-58017-255-5.

Herbal Antibiotics, by Stephen Harrod Buhner. 128 pages. Paperback. ISBN 1-58017-148-6.

Dandelion Medicine, by Brigitte Mars. 128 pages. Paperback. ISBN 1-58017-207-5.

Saw Palmetto for Men & Women, by David Winston. 128 pages. Paperback. ISBN 1-58017-206-7.

Natural First Aid, by Brigitte Mars. 128 pages. Paperback. ISBN 1-58017-147-8.

ADHD Alternatives, by Aviva Romm and Tracy Romm. 128 pages. Paperback. ISBN 1-58017-248-2.

These books and other Storey books are available at your bookstore, farm store, garden center, or directly from Storey Books, Schoolhouse Road, Pownal, Vermont 05261, or by calling 1-800-441-5700. Or visit our Web site at www.storeybooks.com.